THE COMPLETE A–Z GUIDE TO
Good Sex

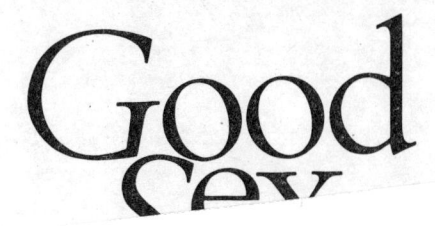

THE COMPLETE A–Z GUIDE TO
Good Sex

Dr. David Delvin

HEREFORD AND WORCESTER
COUNTY LIBRARIES
612.6

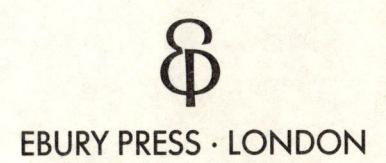

EBURY PRESS · LONDON

First published by Ebury Press
an imprint of the Random Century Group
Random Century House
20 Vauxhall Bridge Road
London SW1V 2SA

1st impression 1990
2nd impression 1991

Copyright © 1990 Dr David Delvin

The right of Dr Delvin to be identified as the author of this work has been asserted by him in accordance with the Copyright, Designs and Patents Act 1988

All rights reserved. No part of the publication may be reproduced, stored in a retrieval system, or transmitted in any form or by any means, electronic, mechanical, photocopying, recording or otherwise, without the prior permission of the copyright owners.

Editor: Viv Croot
Designed by Adrian Morris Publishing Ltd

ISBN 0 85223 919 X

Printed and bound in Great Britain at
the Bath Press, Avon

Love, Relationships, Sex and Sexuality

ADULTERY

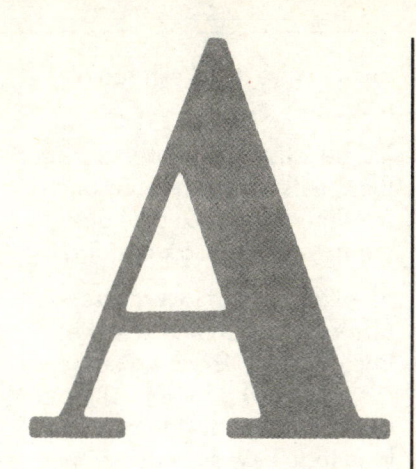

Adultery

'Infants', as somebody once remarked, 'don't have nearly so much fun in infancy as adults do in adultery.' And that's the trouble with adultery. It's awfully tempting – and it always looks as though it would be such fun, and wouldn't do any real harm, would it?

Unfortunately, the trouble is that adultery quite often *does* do harm – to marriages and families, and to people's physical and emotional health.

Of course, it may well lead to divorce. Even today (when adultery is rather less frowned on than it was) about a third of all divorce petitions are brought on grounds of infidelity. In my opinion, the infidelity is usually the *symptom* of problems in marriage rather than their cause.

But there's no doubt that in most cases, if an innocent party finds out about his or her partner's adultery, this is likely to lead to a great deal of emotional upheaval – and sometimes even to violence. The trouble and bitterness may spill over and affect the children of the marriage, something no one in their right mind would want.

You must also bear in mind a couple of simple basic medical

ADULTERY

facts, which are so often forgotten by people who trip down the agreeable primrose path to adultery. First, there may well be a good chance that the affair will result in a woman becoming pregnant by the wrong husband. And secondly, there's always the risk that if your fellow-frolicker in bed is promiscuous, you may wind up with a sexual infection – which you may pass on to your spouse.

Having said all that, I have to admit that people are only human and that they do very often stray from the path of virtue – and frequently get away with it. Adultery is incredibly common these days, even in staid, respectable Britain, it seems likely according to recent surveys that:

three out of 10 wives have committed adultery

half of these have had multiple lovers

at any given time, about one in 10 wives is having an affair.

So if you *are* unwise enough to give in to temptation, what's the best way to manage things and keep the situation from getting out of control? Here are some pointers:

firstly, try to bring the affair to an end if you can – the longer it goes on the more the likelihood of trouble

just because you slipped between the sheets with somebody *once* in a moment of weakness doesn't mean you have to do it again

try at all cost not to turn a sexual affair into a genuine love (i.e. loving) affair. There's a tendency for people who fall into bed out of sheer lust to decide before long that they love each other – and that really can be bad news

laughably simple though it sounds, make sure someone is taking contraceptive precautions. You really are going to mess up a marriage (perhaps two marriages) if it looks as though there's going to be a little cuckoo in the nest

if there's the chance that your frolic might have led to infection then for heaven's sake have a confidential check-up at a clinic. It would be totally unfair to give an infection to your innocent spouse – which often happens

finally, unless there's some really overwhelming reason why you have to, *don't confess*. Few people want to be told that their partner has two-timed them: if you *must* confess to someone, see a priest, doctor or marriage guidance counsellor.

AFFAIRS

Q How can I get myself out of this difficult situation? I have somehow or other drifted into affairs with two men.

The big problem is that they are both 'family'. One is my husband's sister's brother-in-law, and the other is my husband's cousin.

A I suppose that's what they call 'sexual relations', is it?

Seriously, adultery is nearly always a dangerous business. Committing adultery with a man who you're related to is very dangerous. And doing it with TWO men who you're related to is stark raving bonkers!

I don't want to sound unsympathetic, but I'm always a bit baffled by these letters from people who say 'I'm in an unwise sexual liaison; what do I do?'

The only sane course if you're embroiled in a risky adulterous relationship is to stop it right away! In your case, you need to tell both of these blokes that in future, the only crumpet they'll be getting from you will be on the end of a toasting-fork.

Q I am 21, have a young child, and have always enjoyed a good sex life with my husband. But recently he accused me of having an affair, because he claims my vagina has expanded and become too big for him. I have always been faithful to him, so this accusation hurts me.

A I'm sure it does. His idiotic suspicions stem from the common male belief that frequent sexual intercourse enlarges a woman's vagina. This is a ludicrous myth, but you'd be surprised how many men believe it. (There's a well-known 'joke' about a tart who offers to pay a taxi driver by letting him look up her skirt; he eyes her doubtfully, and then says: 'Haven't you got anything smaller?')

Anyway, the only common reason for a vagina being too loose is not lovemaking, but childbirth. I'd suggest you have a check-up from a GP, family planning clinic MO, or gynaecologist, who will tell you whether your vagina needs 'tightening up' with a repair operation, or whether a course of exercise would suffice.

See also **PELVIC FLOOR**

Q What do you think I should do? I am married, but I have somehow slipped into an affair with a man at our local squash club. It all happened when the two of us played a practice

AFFAIRS • ANAL SEX

game together at the club one afternoon. We seemed to get on awfully well on the court, and we laughed together a lot during the game.

There was no-one else in the building at the time. As the men's and the women's changing rooms are next to each other, we continued chatting to one another through the communicating door.

Just after I'd stepped under the shower, I heard him come up behind me. He took me in his arms, and that was that.

Since then, we have gone on making love at the club during the day when it is quiet. Am I mad to go on with this relationship?

A Squash has always had a bit of a reputation as a sexy sort of game. Maybe that's because of the very close physical contact of fairly scantily-dressed men and women in an enclosed space. As the Americans say, 'Nothing propinks like propinquity.'

Also, there's a theory that when males and females perspire, they give off 'pheromones' – scents which are strong sexual attractants, with a powerful effect on the unconscious mind.

Add to all this the heady brew of an 'unchaperoned' building plus adjacent changing rooms and a warm, soapy shower – and you've got a recipe for disaster.

Honestly, ma'am: if you go on meeting this man in this fashion, it's a hundred to one that somebody is going to find out. The news will get to your husband – and to this bloke's wife (if he has one).

So I urge you to join another squash club – or perhaps change to a different sport altogether.

Furthermore, if anybody catches the pair of you in the club showers, your lover is very likely to end up being blackballed (if you'll forgive the phrase).

Q My husband wants me to have anal sex during period times when we can't make love in the ordinary way. But what infections can be passed on?

A Well, AIDS – if, of course, one partner has the HIV virus.

Also, the man can get a urinary infection from the germs in the woman's bowel. And if he were unwise enough to have vaginal intercourse with her immediately afterwards this could give her a vaginal discharge.

Recent work among male gays does suggest that rectal practices, including anal intercourse and kissing ('rimming') do transmit hepatitis, amoebiasis, and an odd form of diarrhoea called 'the gay bowel syndrome'.

Anorgasmia

Anorgasmia means 'inability to reach orgasm', and it is quite common in women, as both my postbag and Dr Kinsey's statistics demonstrate.

Kinsey found that roughly one woman in ten can't reach a climax at all. Many others find considerable difficulty in doing so, and are very worried by this.

But I think that many men and women expect too much of female orgasmic ability.

Many men – especially younger blokes – think that if they have intercourse with a woman, she should automatically and swiftly reach orgasm.

Many younger women think that orgasm should start happening as soon as a girl loses her virginity.

These assumptions are nonsense! Unlike male orgasm, female orgasm isn't almost automatic. It usually needs care, tenderness and skill to produce one – and some women may need an hour or so of stimulation before they are warmed up enough to 'come'.

The ability to reach orgasm is surprisingly low in younger women. According to Kinsey, only about 40% of 20-years-olds can reach an orgasm at all. The ability to have a climax increases rapidly with age, however, and the vast majority of 40-plus women can do it.

So what do you do if you really are having big trouble reaching a climax?

Well, the first thing to clear up is that lack of orgasm is unlikely to have a physical cause and the emotional reasons are many and complex – involving such things as childhood repressions, bad sexual experiences and stress.

One common cause, however, is lack of knowledge. Your man has to know that he is stimulating you in the way that *you* want, and that means you telling him.

Still no luck? Then my advice would be to go to a Family Planning Clinic and ask to see a doctor who has been trained in the 'Balint' or 'Seminar' method of marital therapy. These doctors (mainly women) are adept at helping people unravel the tensions which so often prevent them from reaching orgasm.

An alternative would be to ask your doctor to refer you and your partner to a 'behaviourist' or Masters-Johnson type clinic where the therapists achieve good results in 're-educating', couples who are in difficulties with their sex lives.

Finally, there are a few feminist

ANORGASMIA

groups which attempt to combat anorgasmia through frank mutual 'workshops' and the guided use of self-masturbation and vibrators.

Male anorgasmia

Blokes have this problem too – though nowhere near as commonly as women do. As is the case with most sexual problems, physical causes are uncommon.

However, certain widely-prescribed medications (particularly for high blood pressure) can cause difficulty in reaching orgasm. So too can alcohol.

Men who have had prostate surgery may also experience problems reaching a climax – though here the difficulty is often the fact that the man's ejaculate (that is, his fluid) is 'shot' backwards into his urinary bladder rather than outwards. Unfortunately, nothing much can be done about this – though if the couple want to have children, it is technically possible to collect the sperms from his urine, and then inseminate them into his wife.

A common cause of failure to reach orgasm is simply *tiredness* – often combined with stress. Regrettably, a lot of chaps these days are too proud to admit thay they're a bit too tired (or too uptight) to reach a climax. As a result, we're now seeing the extraordinary new phenomenon of *men* faking orgasm.

Obviously, the remedy in these cases is to try to get to bed earlier. If you're still too tired then, at the end of the day set the alarm for an earlier time than you need in the morning. Alternatively make love out of bed and away from the bedroom which is strongly associated with sleep. Also, be frank with your partner, talk things over with her – and try and relax and take life easier. If these commonsense measures fail, then it's wise to seek professional counselling.

There's a large group of men who suffer from what the Americans have grandly termed 'ejaculatory incompetence'.

They have perfectly normal male hormones, but something (most probably inhibitions from early in life) makes it very difficult for them to actually go over the top and reach orgasm.

They usually enjoy lovemaking, and are often popular with female partners – for the obvious reason that they tend to go on for hours and hours. While this can be pleasurable for the women in their lives, there usually comes a time when a couple decide that 'something's got to be done about it'!

BEREAVEMENT

Bereavement

Unfortunately, one person in virtually every loving couple has eventually to face bereavement from their partner – sometimes tragically early.

If this happens to *you* early in life, it's absolutely devastating. Many people feel like killing themselves – and a few do.

But the fact is that most people who are bereaved early in their married lives do (often much to their amazement) manage to get things back on an even keel. Many of them do eventually start going out with other people – and a lot get married again. Such marriages are often highly successful – though you should *never* rush into one just 'to give the children a father/mother'. As you're doubtless well aware, almost all stepchildren are wary of (and potentially hostile toward) any stepfather or stepmother.

A far more common situation, of course, is for a loving couple to survive 30 or 40 years together, and then to be split up by death quite *late* in life. Though it's common, it doesn't make it easier to bear.

I get a lot of letters from people who've recently been bereaved. The main hope I can offer is

BEREAVEMENT • BISEXUALITY

something every doctor knows: that eventually most of them *do* find a purpose in living, particularly through their interest in their children and grandchildren. Some who have *no* children find fulfilment in helping others.

What about the sexual aspect of bereavement? I receive an amazing number of letters from people who have lost their partners – but who still have very strong sexual feelings. Most of these letters are from women – which is partly a reflection of the fact that women tend to outlive men.

Obviously, it can be very distressing if you're a widow of 65 or 70 and you find that you're still troubled by strong sexual urges (a common situation judging by my postbag). I think the first thing to say is that – in answer to a question frequently raised by grannies (!) who write to my column – yes it's perfectly acceptable to relieve these tensions by masturbation.

However the fact is (however awful it may sound to someone who's recently been bereaved), *you're never too old to get married again*. Many people who've had happy and loving marriages, and who eventually lose their loved ones, do later remarry at 65 or 70. I've even seen people remarry at 90 – which gives one fresh hope, I must say!

Finally, I would like to stress that there is an encouraging new trend in the development of organizations which counsel those who've lost their loved ones. There are bodies like the Compassionate Friends in Britain, or Cruse, who try to help people through the cruel loss of the person they have loved for life.

Q I am under great stress, as I have discovered after 25 years of marriage that my husband has felt the need to find new friends from 'the gay community'. I try to keep the house nice and myself attractive, but I know that he can barely touch me – although I realise that he must have some spark of love left, because he is still very generous with his gifts. Could he be bisexual?

A I'm afraid this is very possible. Indeed, the poor man may have discovered that he's really homosexual, rather than

BISEXUALITY

Bisexuality

Although many people find the whole idea incomprehensible and distasteful, it's undeniable that a good many 'happily married' husbands and wives are bisexual – in other words, they have the urge to obtain sexual pleasure from both men and women.

My eyes were opened to this fact years ago when I worked in a busy VD clinic – where we'd see Mr Jones, respectable banker and father of four, who just *happened* to have a boyfriend in Chelsea. Since then, the bisexual lives of rather a lot of famous people have been revealed, and we've actually reached the extraordinary stage where some pop stars seemed to revel in it.

However, finding that your partner is bisexual is no fun (as Mrs Oscar Wilde discovered). Quite apart from anything else, if the bisexual partner is male there is the everpresent danger of bringing infections – possibly even AIDS – into the home.

Astonishingly though, I have encountered some cases in which a loving spouse was somehow or other willing to make an effort to cope with his or her partner's bisexuality, and make a go of the marriage. This was, of course, the case with the celebrated and eccentric partnership of Harold Nicolson and Vita Sackville-West.

bisexual. I say 'the poor man' because I'm sure he's as distressed as you are by the crisis that has hit your marriage. In fact, this is an increasingly common situation these days: you'd be surprised at the number of husbands who suddenly realise that they're gay. I think that the pair of you have got to come to a decision as to whether you want the marriage to go on. I have known women who made a success of a marriage with a gay or bisexual husband, but it certainly isn't easy. I'm afraid you have to face the fact that a divorce might eventually turn out to be the best solution – especially if, as you say, your husband no longer wants physical contact with you. However, all is not yet lost – there is a 'Relate' Marriage Guidance Clinic in the city from which you write, and I think you should see them – *rapidly*. It'd also be worth getting in touch with the Albany Trust Counselling, *24 Chester Square, London SW1 9JF*, who have great experience in dealing with the social and emotional problems faced by homosexuals – and indeed by the wives of homosexuals.

BONDAGE • THE BOTTOM

Q Your frankness and sense of humour in **SHE** are refreshing, but I really do not understand why you condemn 'kinky' sex games involving bondage.

I am a divorcée with two sons, and we live with my slightly younger boyfriend. My man will sometimes tie me to the bed before making love to me. Or sometimes he will put me across his knee and spank me. I am quite a dominant woman normally, so being 'dominated' in this way can be quite exciting!

A Whatever turns you on, ma'am. All I'm saying is that bondage games do occasionally lead to nasty accidents – which have, on rare occasions, proved fatal. But it doesn't sound as though you two are into anything involving gags, or ropes round the neck.

I also think that women should run a mile if they meet a guy who wants to introduce real sadism into the bedroom. But I do agree with you that your bit of bottom-smacking isn't hurting anyone or anything (except possibly your *derrière*).

The female bottom

The female bottom has always been a subject of great interest to the male sex – as any woman who has ever endured the indignity of a stroll along the Via Veneto will know. But the buttocks are undoubtedly an erogenous zone of the body – so much so that some women can reach orgasm through having their bottoms patted or even slapped. The are so many sexually-tuned nerve endings in that area of the body that a firm stimulus – like gentle slapping – is bound to fire off a few sensual circuits in the nervous system.

It also has to be admitted that the anal area is even more rich with sexually-tuned nerve endings. This is why anal love-play ('postillionage') and even anal intercourse are so common. A *Playboy* sex survey indicated that a rather alarming 54% of those couples who took part in the survey had tried anal sex. I say 'alarming' because of the hygiene risks of this practice.

The male bottom

As with the female bottom, the male one is a sexually arousable area. In other words, most men

THE BOTTOM • BREASTS

like having their buttocks caressed. And as with some women, some men also like having it gently slapped or spanked. With a minority of men, this seems to go a great deal further: in other words, they actually enjoy being caned, even though it hurts a good deal. I cannot account for this male tendency but it seems to be a very widespread one. There may be something in the well known theory that all these men have been deeply influenced by the repeated bottom canings they experienced at school. (But since corporal punishment has become so rare in recent years, it's surprising that the trend has not died out.) There is certainly no harm in a little honest bottom smacking in bed, but there is no point in going in for it unless you really want to.

The other extremely sexual area of the male bottom is the anus. Just as is the case with the female back passage this is a region where there appear to be a lot of erotic nerve endings. A lot of people think that it's only homosexual males who get sexual pleasure in this way but that is not true. In Britain, the USA and many other western countries, it has become the smart thing for sophisticated women to slip a lubricated finger inside the man's rectum while making love, or having oral sex. However, there seem to me to be real risks in doing it, if you're not *very* careful about washing your hands immediately afterwards. In particular, some of the alarming 'new' sexual infections which are spreading across the world may well be transmitted by this sort of play.

Finally, let me add that there is one other quite common way of stimulating the male (or indeed female) bottom. This is with the 'rectal vibrators' which are widely sold in sex shops. I mention these only to say that *you should not use them*. Vaginal vibrators are quite a different thing, but rectal vibrators can sometimes vanish inside you!

Q I have very small breasts. My girl friend wants me to go to a 'non-textile' (ie nudist) beach with her this summer. Do you think I will feel embarrassed?

A Probably. I speak from personal experience — because some time back, I reported on a naturist camp for a medical magazine, and had to strip off to conduct

17

BREASTS

the interviews. However, I can tell you that the embarrassment tends to last about two minutes flat – by which time you've realised that no-one is paying any attention to the size and shape of your personal bits and pieces.

By the bye, I found that naturists were a jolly and friendly lot. They run things like sponsored nude swims in aid of leukaemia. And the organiser of their Singles Club keeps writing to me to say that they need lots more female members. Interested readers should write to CCBN, Assurance House, *35–41 Hazelwood Rd, Northampton NN1 1LL* for a leaflet called Bare With Us!

See also **THE NIPPLE**

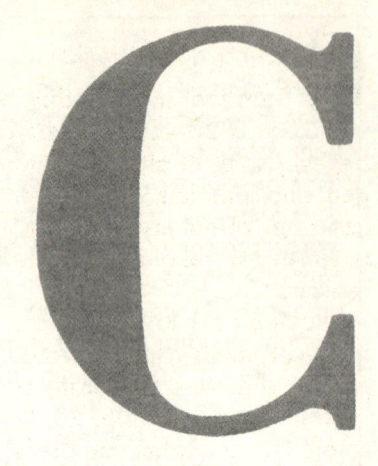

CHILD ABUSE • CLITORAL STIMULATION

Q I am that modern-day rarity, a 23-year-old-virgin. I believe I am an attractive, intelligent and confident woman with no hang-ups about my sexuality. I'm a virgin for religious and moral reasons.

I have a very loving boyfriend, and everything in my life would be perfect, if it were not for my past.

From the age of 14 to 20, I was cajoled by my father into performing various sexual acts with him (I always refused full intercourse). I complied out of love for him, and because I was able to sense his desperation.

He died two years ago, and now I have real emotional happiness with my boyfriend.

My dilemma lies in whether or not I should tell him about my father?

A First of all, I must congratulate you on your immensely courageous letter.

From the unpublished part of it, I gather that you've never told a living soul about your Dad, and feel it would be 'betraying his secret' to talk directly to someone about what he did.

Mainly for that reason, I don't think you should tell your boyfriend – yet. It would be better to kick off by speaking to an anonymous individual, who is experienced in dealing with the problems caused by incest.

So please ring the *Incest Crisis* line – on either 01–422 5100 or 01–890 4732. Their counsellors will, I'm sure, help you lift the burden of the past from your shoulders. Good luck.

Q After 16 years of marriage, my wife has just horrified me by telling me that she wants to rub her own clitoris during intercourse. This has really shaken me.

Should she really *need* this sort of thing?

A Well, I'm sorry if your poor old ego was a bit wounded by your missus' revelation!

But there's no need for alarm. You see, vast numbers of women *do* need clitoral stimulation during sexual intercourse. And my analysis of the returns from a *Delvin Report* shows that many **SHE** readers do actually *give themselves* that stimulation – at the same time as their menfolk make love to them.

Unfortunately, a lot of men just can't handle this (so to speak). But I think you should just regard it as a natural part of your wife's sexuality – and be glad she's happy.

See also **MASTURBATION**

CLITORAL STIMULATION

Clitoral Stimulation

In just the same way as the penis, the clitoris becomes erect during sexual excitement – either as a result of thinking erotic thoughts, or as a result of direct stimulation.

And as is the case with the penis, the clitoris becomes erect simply because it fills up with blood – so that it becomes stiffer.

People do get rather the wrong idea about erection of the clitoris. They've usually read about it in sex manuals or school biology books, and think that the clitoris is going to turn into something like a small courgette!

But in fact your clitoris is a very tiny organ indeed. It's only about the size of a baked bean, and most of it is internal so that from the outside, you can only see a little 'bump' about the size of a shirt button.

Even during sexual excitement, the external part is only about half the size of a processed pea, so that it just peeks out from under the 'hood'.

However, this amount of erection does seem to bring it more firmly into contact with the man's pubic region – which is very important if the woman is to achieve satisfaction.

Q I'm pregnant and find my sexual feelings much stronger than before – I have to rub my clitoris at night. Will this harm the baby?

A Not at all, ma'am particularly as your clitoris is away from where the baby is. If this innocent practice helps you relax and to cope better with your pregnancy – just lie back and enjoy it.

Q Could my umbilicus be connected to my clitoris? My friends think I'm mad, but I wonder if my belly button is an erogenous zone? Certainly, when my fiancé rubs it, I can virtually reach a climax.

A I've heard of naval manoeuvres, but this is ridiculous! If your letter isn't a hoax, then my conclusion is simply that you are remarkably lucky. (And so is your fiancé...)

THE CLITORIS

Clitoris

One of the unexpected bonuses of being lucky enough to have your books translated into foreign languages is that you find out all sorts of useful foreign words.

In German, it's *die Kitzler*, in Dutch its *de clitoris*, in French it's *le cli-cli* and in Hebrew its represented by something that looks like the figures '72727' followed by a picture of Stonehenge.

So there's a lot of interest in the clitoris all over the world. Regrettably, in Britain lots of men and women aren't too clear about just where the clitoris is or what it does. This is a pity, because it is the main key to sexual pleasure in most women.

Because so many couples are vague about the location and function of the clitoris, their sex lives are often frustrating and unhappy. Once they *do* find out where it is – and what to do with it – things often improve dramatically.

A woman's clitoris is located just in front of her pubic bone – so that with a bit of luck, it will be gently compressed and squeezed between the man's pubes and her own during intercourse.

It's only about the same width as a little blouse button – even when it swells up during sexual excitement. But close examination reveals that it is almost identical in structure to a man's penis. So it's not surprising that it's more plentifully supplied with pleasure-producing nerve-endings than any other part of the female body.

I haven't space to embark on description of the many possible clitoris-stimulation techniques. But male readers may like to note the point that during love-play, many lasses (not all) do prefer to be stimulated along the *side* of the clitoris, rather than directly on top of it.

Disorders of the clitoris are rare. Occasionally women seek medical advice because of a sudden and alarming swelling of the clitoris. This swelling appears to be due to a collection of blood – and it soon bursts, leaving no ill-effects.

Some years ago, I described the condition in the doctors' magazine *World Medicine*, and promptly received a number of letters from practitioners who had seen it. Two of them mentioned cases in which the woman had actually caused the swelling by wrapping a cotton thread round her clitoris during masturbation – clearly, this is *not* a sensible idea.

CONDOMS • CONDOM ALLERGY

Q Help, help, help! My fiancé and I have been using the condom as our means of contraception, but we've had three of the said objects burst on us! I thought that these wonderful 'AIDS-preventing' condoms had stringent tests?

A They do, they do – not only electronic tests but also being filled with water and being dropped from a great height!

However, the fact is that the public (both male and female) like condoms to be sensitive – and that means very thin indeed. So inevitably, there will be times when even a completely flawless condom will tear.

You can minimise the chances of this happening by:

(a) following the instructions on the manufacturer's leaflet to the letter (or even the French letter).
(b) Taking great care to avoid nicking the sheath with fingernails, engagement rings – or even teeth.

But if the condoms continue to burst, it could be due to the fact that your fiancé is ... er ... a very big lad. In which case you may possibly wish to switch to another method. (British manufacturers do not make specially big condoms – they're all one size).

One final point for all condom-users out there. The Family Planning Association does recommend that women protect themselves against the risk of a burst condom by using a vaginal spermicidal pessary as well. You can buy these without embarrassment at chemist's – and in Family Planning Clinics, where they're usually given out in the same pack as the condoms.

Condom Allergy

There's good news for those couples who can't use sheaths because of an allergy. Durex have launched a new, lubricated hypo-allergenic sheath, simply (if unimaginatively) called 'Durex Allergy'.

I must say that if I were a bloke who had an allergy to French letters, I'd certainly prefer these new condoms to the alternative answer, which is to use a sheath made not of rubber, but of lambs' intestines (yuk).

CROSS DRESSING

Q I'm due to be married next Easter, and my fiancé has just told me he likes dressing up in women's clothes. What do I do?

A I'm sure this has come as a big shock to you. But there are many 'cross-dressers' around. Rather surprisingly, quite a lot of them do make happy and successful marriages – though their wives have to be pretty understanding.

One possible factor in the success of some of these marriages is that quite a few women do seem to get a kick out of seeing men dressed up in women's clothing, though I don't know why.

But I think you must go very carefully during the next few months. Talk this over very thoroughly with your fiancé before you agree to go ahead with the wedding. You *must* ask him whether he has homosexual or bisexual leanings – though in fact, many transvestites are basically heterosexual.

Even if you love the guy very much, I think you might do better to live with him for a while, before you actually tie the nuptial knot with someone who may be borrowing your knickers for the next 60 years. Good luck.

Cross Dressing

Most people assume that because transvestites like dressing up in 'drag', they must be homosexual. But the spokesperson for their organisation says that nearly all the gents who belong to his society are very much heterosexual – and often married too.

I'm inclined to believe him. Some years ago, the medical journal for which I work despatched a woman reporter to cover a conference for transvestite men.

Afterwards, she indignantly reported that one of them had tried to grope her in the back of a taxi – despite the fact that he was wearing diamanté earrings and evening gown!

DIVORCE

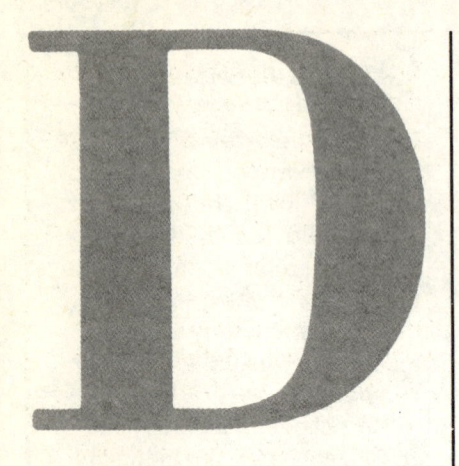

Q I am a divorcée, heading for 40, lonely but still quite attractive. Last summer I went on a sailing holiday in Greece and much to my surprise had a tremendously satisfying affair with a young Greek courier.

Now he has written to me, inviting me to come sailing with him this summer in the Aegean. Do you think I'd be crazy to renew this relationship with a man who is about half my age?

A I don't think you'd be crazy at all, ma'am. Sailing in Greece provides a tremendous holiday (even if – like Cap'n Delvin last year – you very nearly scuppered your yacht in the wine-dark sea!).

If you, as a lonely, 40-ish divorcée, can combine a sailing holiday in that beautiful country with a satisfying emotional and physical relationship provided by some young Apollo, then good luck to you.

One shouldn't always beware the Greeks when they come bearing (or indeed, baring) gifts...

Divorce

It's a pretty awful thought that (in most western societies) at least one in three of all those who get married will some day have to face marriage breakdown.

It's tragic, but those are the facts. I get more and more depressed when I read the divorce statistics each year!

Although there are variations between countries, it seems that almost everywhere, the trend towards divorce is on the increase. Repeated divorce – or 'serial monogamy', as they call it in California, has now become quite socially acceptable.

Britain is fairly typical of most western societies: 80% of all divorces occur in first marriages. Which means, if you think about it, that one in five of all divorces involves somebody for whom this was already the second marriage!

Indeed, in nearly one in 10 cases, *both husband and wife* have been married before, and are going through their second divorce. This lends new weight to Dr Johnson's famous statement that second marriages represent 'a triumph of hope over experience'!

Obviously, I can only hope to deal in this book with the sexual side of coping with a divorce. But if divorce does strike your marriage, how are *you* going to cope with it sexually?

The first thing to say is this. *Don't assume that your love-life is over*!

Although I've said that a second marriage should be regarded with caution, there's no reason to feel that matrimony is 'out' for you from now on.

Nor are enjoyable romantic relationships with the opposite sex by any means over. It's very easy for a divorced person – particularly a woman – to think, "My love-life is finished.' But that's not necessarily true: life still holds plenty of romance – and *divorcées* (and *divorcés* too) are socially very much in demand these days!

Indeed, the problem for both *divorcée* and *divorcé* may be quite the reverse. Enthusiastic would-be lovers tend to swarm round any recently divorced person who is even half-way attractive, and there may be very real difficulty in keeping all these characters out of your bed!

I have to say that there's a terrible tendency among many newly-divorced people (both men and women) to give in to the temptation to partake 'not wisely, but too well' of all these

DIVORCE

offers. I have received in my postbag a fairly typical letter from a recently-divorced woman who had been quite 'bowled over' to find out, after all these years of monogamy, that she was highly attractive to men.

The poor lady had (according to her letter) slept with all the handsome men who flocked round her, and had (I quote) 'a fantastic time', as she discovered that most of them were far better lovers than her husband. This experience is common.

Unfortunately, in the end (literally) she got herpes. Naturally, she was now pretty distraught. She'd been particularly distressed at the idea that she'd 'never be able to make love again' – which fortunately isn't really true.

This kind of wild over-indulgence often occurs after divorce. It may result in:

sexual infection

emotional hurt

unwanted pregnancy

difficulties with existing children – who may understandably be very upset that a parent keeps coming home with a replacement Daddy or Mummy on Saturday nights.

So, play it a bit cool. *Don't rush headlong into unwise affairs.* *Do remember that contraception is (usually) still necessary.* *Do remember that one-night stands tend to bring infection.* And above all, bear in mind that *you must not let your love-life upset your children.*

However, never forget that you do still have a chance of finding a life-long loving relationship. Despite Sam Johnson's dictum about repeat marriages, they do very often succeed. Why, you've only to look at Ronald Reagan and Nancy!

EJACULATION

Q I have been told that for a man to 'hold back' when he feels ejaculation coming on is dangerous and may cause internal injury, is this true?

A No, I think this is a myth. There was a time when certain naturopaths used to suggest that 'holding back' could cause enlargement of the prostate in later life. But there's no medical evidence whatever for this.

In practice, it would be very difficult for a man to be any kind of a decent lover unless he learned to postpone his climax, in order to prolong his partner's enjoyment.

Q My boyfriend has asked me to write to you about the subject of female ejaculation, because he says you know about it.

I thought I was abnormal when I first did it at a climax, and felt terribly ashamed. But he says it is normal. Is this true? And if so, what is the fluid which I produce at the moment of orgasm?

A Your boyfriend is quite right. Surprisingly, it's normal for some women to squirt out a fluid at the

EJACULATORY INCOMPETENCE

moment of orgasm. This usually causes them great distress until they eventually find out that it's OK.

Along with most other docs, I used to believe that this fluid was always urine – and that the ladies were being slightly incontinent under the wholly understandable stress of 'coming'!

But research in America has suggested very strongly that it's actually a special sex fluid, rather similar to the secretion which is ejaculated from a man's prostate gland, but produced by a sensitive structure near the famous G-spot. (That G-spot gets everywhere these days, doesn't it?)

Actually, I'm not yet totally convinced by the US research on the chemical nature of this liquid, but (as far as I know) no-one this side of the Atlantic has tried to analyse it.

A **SHE** reader did once attempt to send me a sample of her fluid, but most unfortunately the bottle broke in the post with disastrous results!

See also **THE G-SPOT; ORGASM; THE VAGINA**

Q You seem to get quite a lot of letters about premature ejaculation. Well, my husband's trouble is the opposite. **In fact, he simply cannot 'come'. He can have sex with me, but during the five years we've been together, he has only ejaculated twice.**

On those two occasions he only managed it after a marathon effort of interminable 'bonking', which was very sore and painful for me.

A Sorry to hear about this. Your husband's problem is called 'ejaculatory incompetence', and there's quite a bit of it about. Cause is unknown, but thought to be emotional.

Happily, the old behaviourist firm of Masters and Johnson have a system of 're-training' which usually does the trick. It would involve you – and you'd need to be prepared to spend many hours in the type of activity usually undertaken by topless masseuses.

Not all wives are willing to do this but your letter gives me the impression that you are keen to help your man overcome (sorry) his disability.

Now you need a therapist to teach you both the re-training programme. Please give the Family Planning Service a ring on 01-636-7866, and they'll be able to give you the nearest one.

See also **ANORGASMIA**

ENGAGEMENT • ERECTION

Engagement

Being engaged can be either a very happy or a very difficult time. Unfortunately, there are often stresses from all sides – from parents, relatives, friends and (if it's a second marriage – as it often is these days) from former wives and/or husbands!

There are also difficult financial pressures – unless you're very rich! There can be tricky social obligations, with the need to keep all sorts of people happy.

And there's the major stress (at least, it's a major stress for a lot of people) of having to be the central actors in that emotion-charged theatrical event: a wedding. No wonder so many brides (and grooms) do a bunk.

The important things to remember during an engagement:
1. Be patient with your partner – because he or she is probably under a lot of stress too.
2. Be nice to your partner's family (even if it's the ex-wife or ex-husband!). The family bitterness that so frequently arises at or before a wedding will all too often last a lifetime.
3. If you become doubtful about marriage, *for heaven's sake put it off!* It doesn't matter what arrangements have been made or how much money will be lost (it doesn't even matter if you're pregnant): the fact is that you should never embark on the frail ship of matrimony unless you're absolutely *sure* that this is the sailor you want to spend the rest of the voyage with. Because the rest of the voyage is *life*.
4. Similarly, if the two of you seem to be sexually incompatible – or if one or other of you has serious sex problems – then think very carefully before going ahead with the wedding. Far too many people think that 'it'll be all right when we're married.' It probably won't.

Q Sex with my husband is super, but – embarrassingly for him – he does tend to lose his erection a little, about half way through intercourse. Is there anything we can do about this?

A A common problem, ma'am. In fact, there's a simple solution, providing the difficulty is relatively mild.

Next time you're making love with him, slip your hand down

ERECTION

Erection

The function of erection is rather vital to the survival of the human race.

First of all, can I make the point that it's important for women to realise that most men tend to be a bit obsessed with this particular human function. Which is not surprising, really – because it's very difficult and frustrating and embarrassing for a bloke if erection doesn't happen when wanted.

The actual stiffening of the penis is caused by a dramatic increase in blood flow into the three hollow chambers which make up most of the organ.

But what makes the male organ become engorged with blood like this? It's a complicated interaction between three different areas of the human nervous system, one of which has been discovered by Professor Julia Polak and her colleagues at Hammersmith Hospital.

This new area of the nervous system works by releasing a chemical with the unlikely name of VIP (it stands for vasoactive intestinal polypeptide.)

Research in Britain, Denmark and France shows that some impotent men are lacking in VIP and if you inject it into a man's penis, he will develop an erection. So there are some hopes that it'll eventually be possible to manufacture the stuff as a cure for impotence.

However, under ordinary circumstances, there are two different factors which will give a man an erection. They are (a) thinking about sex (b) direct rubbing or stroking of his penis.

It seems that in some way, these activities release the above-mentioned VIP into the man's phallus, and to help make it erect.

Now it's absolutely vital for any woman to realise that activity (a) above – ie 'thinking about sex' – may well not be enough to give a male an erection, particularly if he's nervous or tired, or perhaps not quite as young as he was.

Yes – contrary to what you might think from reading certain popular novels, quite a few men don't 'leap to attention' as soon as their beloved starts taking her clothes off!

So the point I'm making is that many chaps do need quite a lot of activity (b), mentioned above, before they're in a fit state to make love.

So there it is, dear readers: very often the future of your man's potency is quite literally in your hands . . .

ERECTION • EXERCISE AND SEX

between your two tums (so to speak) and hold him, firmly but agreeably, stimulating with your fingers as necessary.

If more wives knew this simple ploy, far fewer gents would have probs with potency.

Q I'm 67, and my husband is 70, and he's having trouble satisfying me these days. This is because his erection is so unreliable.

Are there any drugs (private or NHS) which would enable him to become erect, even if it was only once or twice a month?

A Yes, there are now. But I must stress that your husband ought to talk this problem over carefully with your doc – and have a physical examination – before any decision is made as to whether to use these VERY powerful drugs. They have to be injected directly into the penis just before sex, and they can have rather drastic side-effects (like, for instance, an erection that simply won't go down unless a surgeon removes blood from the engorged organ).

For that reason, the injection treatment is as a rule prescribed by urological surgeons, rather than by GPs.

Exercise and Sex

Recently there have been persistent suggestions in the newspapers that exercise is somehow bad for you sexually. But what are the facts?

Well, earlier this year I was fortunate enough to chair a sports medicine symposium at which one of the speakers was medical officer to the British women's team in a certain sport. (For obvious reasons, I won't say *which* sport...)

He revealed that the intensive training which these international sportswomen go in for has one little-known side-effect. Virtually none of them have periods.

It appears that heavy and repeated exercise (for instance, running 50 or so miles a week is likely to stop a woman's periods. Some top sports-women haven't had 'the curse' for years.

Fortunately, the effect seems to be only *temporary*, and it's thought that most sportswomen get their periods back when they stop training.

And what about their love-lives? As far as I can discover, although many top sportswomen don't menstruate they still have a perfectly healthy interest in sex. A high proportion feel it wisest to take the pill (since the absence of

EXERCISE AND SEX

periods *doesn't* mean that you can't get pregnant).

Indeed, it's rumoured that in a recent British women's sports team, every member but one was on the pill. The odd one out turned out to be a man.

What about the effect of exercise on *blokes'* sex lives?

I've noticed a lot of reports in the media which claim that jogging causes impotence. Indeed, when I was doing a radio phone-in recently I was *assured* by the presenter that this anti-erotic effect of jogging had been proved by an American university. 'They've shown that it lowers your male hormone levels' he told me.

Well I've got good news for anxious joggers. In fact, the whole thing was an April Fools' Day hoax in my own medical newspaper *General Practitioner*!

Unfortunately, the hoax was swallowed hook, line and sinker by a national paper, and it's been constantly repeated since then.

But I can assure you, gents – the only way that jogging will make you limp is if you twist your ankle!

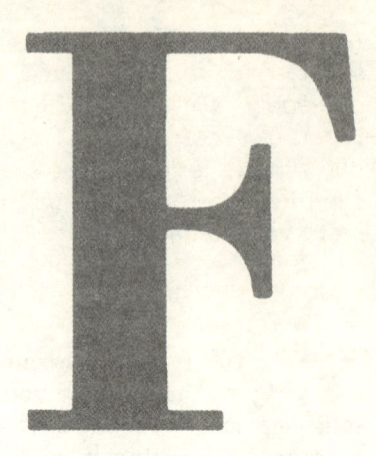

FOREPLAY • FOURSOMES

Q For how long are men supposed to provide women with foreplay?

I ask because I really am getting rather tired of providing this service for my wife. Sometimes she wants as much as 15 minutes before I'm allowed to have intercourse with her.

A Well sir, I've recently come across an American sex survey in which a large number of US ladies were asked: 'How long do you usually like loveplay to last?'

The answers (which may shatter you somewhat) were as follows:

less than five minutes	2 per cent
five to fifteen minutes	36 per cent
up to half an hour	48 percent
up to an hour	14 per cent

So, many women prefer up to 30 minutes of love play – and some want up to an hour. Your poor old missus is being relatively undemanding in only asking for up to 15 minutes.

Frankly, the general tone of your question is so selfish that it makes me a bit dubious about the prospects for your marriage. I suggest you rapidly review your attitude to your wife's sexual and emotional needs – before she starts looking for love play elsewhere.

See also **LOVE PLAY**

Q I read what you said about the survey that showed so many women wanted lots of foreplay.

Now I really think I'm odd, because I don't like it at all. I'm 38, and happily married with a great sex life. But I like to get right on with it! I hate being petted first. Am I the only one!

A Not at all, ma'am. It looks as though about a few per cent of women are satisfied with less than five minutes of loveplay before intercourse. And a substantial number of them simply can't stand foreplay at all, and just want to get right on with it – like you.

Indeed, marital arts specialists find that when these women come into the consulting room complaining about their sex lives, the best thing to do is to tell their husbands to abandon all attempts at preliminary petting and just charge right in!

Q I just don't know what to do about my marriage. Several years ago, my wife and I drifted into a foursome with a very nice couple who share our interests in chamber music, opera,

FOURSOMES • FRUSTRATION

bridge, ski-ing – and of course sex.

No one else knew that the four of us had this sexual arrangement, and it all seemed very discreet and civilised. But things began to go wrong when we all went ski-ing in Kitzbühl last winter. To be frank, the two wives seemed to get more and more interested in each other, and less and less interested in us.

By the time we came home, they appeared to be very emotionally wrapped up in one another. And now both of them seem to have lost all interest in their marriages, and they are talking about setting up home together.

Have you any suggestions as to what we two husbands should do?

A I'm sorry to hear about this predicament, but I'm not surprised.

In Britain there's been a very strong trend toward these 'discreet' and 'civilised' mixed foursomes ever since the 1960s. Some couples have got away with such arrangements, but many others have hit serious troubles.

What usually happens is that the wife in marriage A falls in love with the husband in marriage B and they go off together, with resultant chaos all round.

Various permutations are possible, but I must admit that your particular situation (with the two wives falling in love with each other during the warm glow of the *après ski*) is a trifle unusual.

So what are you to gents to do? If both your wives are basically lesbian, then I think you've had it.

But I reckon that there's a chance you might be able to win them back if you're willing to try really hard.

This means devoting yourself to trying to romance your wife, and to wooing her back to you single-mindedly. Make clear to her that you love her, and that you'd give anything to have her back again.

Most important of all, tell her that from now on, you want her one-to-one, and not with some other bloke sharing the goodies. Then for heaven's sake, bid this other couple farewell – and don't get involved in any more sexual shenanigans with them.

Q I'm not a nymphomaniac but I do need sex very badly. If I don't get it, I become very edgy.

But I split up from my boyfriend some time back. So what do I do? I refuse to 'sleep around' just to relieve my frustration until Mr Right happens to come along!

A I entirely agree with you. For a highly sexed woman such as

FRUSTRATION

yourself, it is much more sensible and safe to rely on masturbation until the right relationship eventually turns up.

Don't feel bad about doing this! One **SHE** survey suggested that a staggering 85 per cent of readers sometimes go in for a spot of 'DIY'. So you'd be in good company, so to speak.

Q I have a good relationship with my husband. However, just after my period finishes each month, I feel very sexually aroused, and want to make love to my husband. Unfortunately, he doesn't share this feeling. He says I'm putting him under pressure, so that he feels like a 'performing animal'. So he just won't reciprocate. This makes me upset and angry, which makes him retreat even more. What can I do?

A Difficult. If this only happens just at the end of your period, I'd say that he's probably one of the many men who aren't totally happy with the fact that women actually menstruate. (The ancient male taboos against having sex with 'menstruous women' are very strong — see the Book of Leviticus). But I think it's more likely that he can't cope with being 'hunted' rather than the 'hunter'.

Either way, I reckon that you both need to sort this out quickly — or your marriage could be heading into trouble. Ask him if he'll go along with you for a chat at 'Relate'; you'll find them in the phone book probably still under their old name — the Marriage Guidance Council.

Q My husband is away in the Merchant Navy for months at a time, and to be frank I get very frustrated sexually.

Recently I have discovered to my surprise that I can ease this frustration by gently playing my hair dryer over my 'pubes'.

Have you any medical objection to this?

A None at all. Better a blow-dry than a boyfriend.

THE G-SPOT

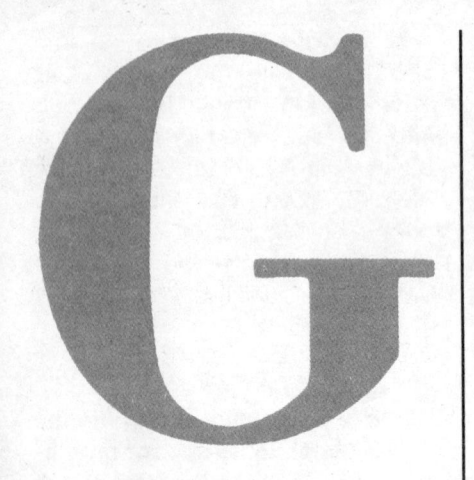

The G-spot

Controversy still rages about whether the 'magic female G-spot' really exists or not. I am inclined to think that it *does* – and that stimulation of it can help some women who have difficulty in getting sexually aroused, or in reaching a climax. It may also be connected with the curious phenomenon of 'female ejaculation'.

My knowledge of the G-spot goes back to a time several years ago when I wrote in my column that it was a 'complete myth' that women ejaculated a fluid at the moment of orgasm. I was immediately flooded with protest letters from readers who said that they *did* do this. One lady even sent

Q Where on earth is my blooming G-spot?

My husband and I have tried repeatedly to find it, but no luck at all. We gather it's half-way up the front wall of the vagina, but we just seem to get a bit lost.

Could you print a map?

A Well ma'am, I'm still a bit doubtful whether the Famous Female G-spot really exists – but

THE G-SPOT

me a sample of the liquid, but the container broke in the post.

At this stage, two readers wrote to me to point out that an obscure US sexological journal had just published a series of research papers which indicated that women had something called a G-spot (named after its discoverer, Ernst Grafenberg), and that stimulation of this newly-discovered organ could produce a climax – a climax which was sometimes accompanied by a squirt of some mysterious sexual fluid.

It's located in very much the same situation as the male prostate gland, and it's interesting that US and Canadian researchers have claimed that the liquid which it's supposed to produce is in fact very similar in chemical composition to the secretion of the prostate. So it's claimed that the 'G-spot' is a sort of 'homologue' (i.e. an exact anatomical equivalent) of a man's prostate gland.

Not altogether surprisingly, the new 'anti-sex movement' in the USA has been claiming that the G-spot doesn't exist at all. But whether it does or not, searching for it may actually help some women with sexual difficulties. If you or partner gently rub an area about half-way up the front wall of your vagina with a soft fingertip, you'll rapidly be able to draw your own conclusions as to whether the G-spot is real – or just a fig-leaf of somebody's imagination...

I'm inclined to think that there's *something* there, if you can only put your finger on it....

It is claimed that the G-spot is a specially sensitive female organ – the exact equivalent of the male prostate gland.

American sexperts claim that stimulation of it helps women who have difficulty reaching orgasm – and that the climaxes produced by rubbing this spot are more intense than ordinary ones – and may be accompanied by release of some special love-fluid.

My own feeling is that the G-spot may not be a real organ at all – but just a very sensitive area over the urethra (water-pipe) – which is just in front of the vagina.

But how the heck do you find it? Best thing is to wait until love-play has you well-lubricated. Then lie on your tummy on the bed, with your legs well apart.

Your husband should sit beside you, and should gently slip his index and middle fingers into your vagina (palm downwards).

He'll find that he can sort of

THE G-SPOT • GROUP SEX

'hook' the pads of his fingertips over the shelf-like projection of your pubic bone. Just beyond this is the area of your G-spot. It's undeniable that if he caresses this zone with his fingers, you will experience all sorts of agreeable and unusual sensations.

Well, that's the G-plan! I hope you're all joining in at home...

Q Am I abnormal? You see, I read what you said about the 'magic G spot'. I appear to have *five* of these in my vaginal area, all very sexually excitable.

A Lucky old you. No, you're not abnormal. Lots of people have more than one specially sensitive area inside their vagina.

Group Sex

Group sex is very popular these days: you'd be amazed how many discreet orgies are arranged in well-appointed London town houses, or in 'respectable' Californian ranch houses. But everything I've said about the dangers of wife-swapping and open marriages applies with about 50 times more force to group sex.

For a start, the multiplicity of sexual contacts in a single evening is just an open invitation to germs to have a ball (if you'll pardon the expression). When I worked regularly at a London VD clinic, I used to see men who had ...er... 'embraced' 25 ladies the previous Saturday night – and who now had to telephone these 25 ladies (and their husbands) to tell them that they urgently needed to go to a clinic for a check-up.

Quite seriously, outbreaks of thrush, gonorrhoea and NSU, of jealousy and even of violence have forced the activities of many wife-swapping circles to grind – so to speak – to a halt.

If AIDS gets a hold among the devotees of wife-swapping orgies (as it has among the *gay* orgy set), then the results could be monumentally disastrous.

IMPOTENCE

Impotence

Let's be quite clear that virtually every man has difficulty in 'making it' at some time in his life. Occasional episodes of this sort are nothing to worry about, and the important thing is that both partners should just do their best not to make a big deal of it!

But it's a different situation when a man keeps on and on having trouble with his potency. This can sap his confidence and ruin his relationship with his partner.

Now why does impotence occur? It's usual to say that some cases are physical, but that most are emotional in origin. But – as a leading article in the *British Medical Journal* recently pointed out – in many men, it is a mixture of the two.

For example, there may be a slight physical problem which sometimes makes it difficult for a man to get a good erection. But he reacts to this with panic and (let's say) his wife reacts to it with scorn, then – bingo – there's now an enormous emotional problem as well.

The average bloke finds it difficult to see how his emotions can make him impotent. But to understand, this we have to look at the mechanisms which cause erec-

IMPOTENCE

tion in the human male. I'm sorry to say that these are not completely understood by us docs yet, but broadly speaking, what we do know is this.

Erection happens when blood is suddenly pumped into cavities inside the man's penis. Some sort of valve mechanism seems to stop the blood from flowing out again while he remains sexually excited.

But what causes these extraordinary hydraulic changes in a chap's John Thomas? Basically, they're caused by impulses which flow along the nerves which control the penile blood vessels.

One powerful set of impulses is generated if you stroke your man's penis. This simple action should fire off a spinal reflex which tells the blood vessels to start pumping blood into his male organ.

Another powerful set originates in his brain. If he starts thinking about you in a sexy way, this should send signals down his spine, and into the nerves which lead to the penile blood vessels.

Unfortunately, the chemical mechanism by which all these impulses are sent to his penis is incredibly complex and delicate. And nervousness, tension, depression and even tiredness can block them.

So that's why the emotions play an important part in impotence.

However, there can be physical factors too. Alcohol is the most common of these. Other drugs can also play a part – and these include several of the pills which are widely used for treating high blood pressure. Abuse of 'hard' drugs is also a notorious cause of impotence. While a man's on heroin or cocaine, for example, he's very likely to find he's off the boil sexually.

Actually physical diseases don't commonly cause impotence. But erection difficulties are variously associated with diabetes, disorders of the nerve tissues and with 'hardening of the arteries'.

Hormone deficiencies rarely cause impotence. But being *fat* increases the chances – and slimming down may sometimes put things right.

What all this adds up to I'm afraid, is that there isn't often a simple and easy answer to the problem of impotence. I wish there were a pill which would immediately cure the millions of blokes who are impotent – but there isn't at the moment.

However, a distinguished woman doctor at the Hammersmith Hospital is working on a

IMPOTENCE

chemical which might lead to a 'potency pill'.

But in the meantime, what can be done if your fella is impotent? Get him to see a doc, in order to rule out the above-mentioned physical causes. A brief physical examination, plus a couple of blood tests, should be sufficient to sort this out.

Almost invariably, you're then left to face the fact that the problem is basically an emotional one. This is nothing for either of you to be ashamed of. In today's crazy, stress-ridden world, it's not surprising that so many men are too tense, too anxious, too tired or too unhappy to make love!

It's terribly important that you – as his loving partner – should do your best to make him feel both relaxed and wanted at bedtime. Whether he recovers will depend greatly on how much *you* can build up his (probably rather shaken) self-esteem.

Probably the most successful therapists where impotence is concerned are the *behaviourists*, and especially those who practice the famous 'Masters and Johnson' method of therapy. This mainly involves in-depth counselling followed by the 'forbidding' of attempts at intercourse, plus encouragement of non-demanding physical activity between the couple, in a relaxed atmosphere. Dotty though it sounds, this does take 'pressure to perform' off the man – and in an encouraging number of cases, it leads to restoration of potency.

I want to conclude by telling you about one or two slightly more dramatic remedies, some of which offer considerable hope for the future.

However, I do want to emphasise that some of these methods of treatment are still largely experimental. And the results which they can achieve are pretty uncertain.

However, there is one well-tried, low-risk method. It's called 'desensitisation therapy', and it's particularly useful for men whose impotence is caused by anxiety. (Nervousness just at the moment of attempting penetration is a very common cause of sudden collapse of a gent's erection.)

Desensitisation therapy works thus. The man lies on a couch while his therapist encourages him to fantasise about the moment of penetration.

As his nervousness rises, the therapist uses techniques based on pyschotherpay to help him relax. The therapist may even inject small doses of a sedative

IMPOTENCE • INFIDELITY

drug into a vein as the patient reports that his anxiety is increasing. This 'titration of tranquillisation against anxiety' can sometimes be quite helpful in helping a chap overcome the nerves which have been undermining his potency.

Much more drastic is the new technique of injecting certain drugs directly into the penis when you want to have intercourse.

This is still very controversial, but some good results have been reported after injecting with alpha-symphathetic blockers – drugs which affect the nerves which control erection.

But there can be problems. The injection can produce a very prolonged and painful erection, which simply won't go dowm. This can be dangerous.

Also, it's not really practical to keep a doctor in the bedroom to give you a jab in the penis whenever you want to make love. A few specialists have got round this problem by training the man's partner to give the intrapenile injection – but a jab wrongly-aimed by an amateur can be very risky. (I must say, the introduction of this therapy does lend new meaning to the phrase 'Just a little prick . . . ')

Finally, it's sometimes possible for a surgeon to insert a splint. Nowadays this can be inflatable, pumped up when needed.

Q I don't really mind, but I've just discovered that my husband had a 'massage' while away on business in Hong Kong. Is this sort of thing common?

A I'm afraid so, ma'am. Your letter seems to indicate that you've decided to forgive him – and I hope he appreciates that fact.

I do feel sorry for the wife (above) who discovered that her husband had a quick 'massage' while on a business trip to 'Ong Kong. Most women are probably quite unaware that nowadays businessmen and other male travellers constantly have this temptation put in front of them (so to speak).

There are very few major cities you can go to without encountering ads for massage services. Very often, they're a prominent feature of the brochures which are left in your hotel room.

One can't exactly approve of this sort of thing, but I suppose it is at least preferable to prostitution, with its terrible attendant dangers

INFIDELITY

of VD and other infections (not to mention the appalling risk of pregnancy of unknown-origin for the prostitute).

Anyway, I'm fascinated to note that in the massage area too, equality of the sexes is creeping in. Yes: one or two London magazines are now actually carrying ads in which gents offer 'visiting massage' to women.

> LADIES ONLY. Visiting massage service. Tuesday, Wednesday and Thursday only. Des will relax you.

Eager to investigate this new anti-sexist trend, I asked a lady colleague to reply to one of these small ads (*not* the one above). She received a very nice letter from a chap called Leon – who is apparently only too willing to provide tired businesswomen with relaxing body massage.

I'm glad to say that my female colleague didn't take him up on his offer – but she was impressed by the fact that Leon is so devoted to his work that he provides his visiting service free of charge!

Infidelity

Unfortunately, we have to face the fact that infidelity is very common. Various US and British surveys have suggested that as many as 50% of all husbands are unfaithful to their wives at some time.

And recent surveys in the USA and Britain have now confirmed that infidelity is alarmingly common in women too. For instance, studies carried out on the readers of what are generally thought of a highly respectable and conservative women's magazines indicate that at least three out of 10 wives have been unfaithful.

These studies are open to one major criticism, and it's this: women who have very strict and puritanical moral views *tend to refuse to take part in such surveys*, whereas women who are very 'easy-going' sexually are likely to have few inhibitions about answering the questions. So this factor may, of course, artificially inflate the apparent proportion of wives who have been unfaithful to their partners.

Nonetheless, any doctor or marriage guidance counsellor will tell you that it's very common to have to cope with a person who's terribly distraught because he or she has found out about his or her partner's infidelity.

This section isn't about adultery. It's about *how to cope with your partner's adultery*.

43

INFIDELITY

So how *are* you going to cope with it? Well, the old ways of 'coping' with infidelity was to set about divorcing your partner immediately – or possibly to make arrangements for shooting them.

That really doesn't seem awfully sensible these days. If *everyone* divorced (or, indeed, shot) his or her spouse solely because of infidelity, there wouldn't be that many marriages left (and rather a lot of bodies around, too).

There's no doubt that finding out that your partner has been unfaithful can be a very shattering experience. Unless you're running some sort of 'open-marriage' you're likely to be extremely upset – to say the least.

In the past, I've seen quite a few women and men who've simply never recovered from the shock of their spouse's infidelity: many years later, they're still depressed and resentful.

But, if you're going to make a go of your marriage, then clearly you have to try and react in a more positive way than this, difficult though it may be.

Here are a few basic suggestions as to how you might deal with the situation:

although it may be terribly hard, try to be generous-minded; have a blazing row if you wish, but always keep in your mind the possibility of forgiveness

think coolly and clearly about just how common such silly affairs are

once you've vented your feelings, try to think about the *temptations* which have made your partner go astray. (Was it during a business trip abroad by one of you? Was she or he lonely and fed up when sudden and seductive 'consolation' – in the shape of sex – was offered?)

painful though it may be, try to think about what *you* have done which might have pushed your partner towards infidelity. (If you don't think you've ever done anything like that, you must indeed be a remarkable and saintly person!)

think particularly about whether you've been tender and loving enough recently

think about whether you've been understanding and sympathetic, and whether you've listened to your partner's problems and worries and tried to help her or him

think about whether you've made yourself *attractive* enough to your partner lately – banal though it sounds, the fact is that

INFIDELITY

again and again, people go off and have sex with somebody else because their own partner has let her – or himself go. I wish I had £10 for every time I've heard a really unwashed and scruffy-looking person saying 'I just can't understand why she/he did it . . .'

finally, think about whether you've taken the trouble to be *sexually pleasing* enough to your partner recently. Again, that sounds trite: yet time and again, wives take lovers because their husbands won't make love to them often enough; or husbands go with other women because their wives aren't sexually adventurous enough in bed.

I know that what I've said will irritate many people, because it puts so much responsibility on the *innocent* party. But if you want to keep the marriage going, then clearly *both* of you (not just the guilty party) have got to work hard at it.

Two final 'no-nos': firstly, don't respond to your partner's infidelity by confessing some past unfaithfulness of your own (if you've had one) – still less by flinging it in his or her face!

Why not? Studies indicate that human beings (i.e. people like your partner) are so idiotic that they tend to regard their own infidelities as 'not very important' – but they tend to regard their spouse's affairs as 'very serious indeed'!

So resist the urge to shriek 'Well – *now* I can tell you that you're not the only one: I did it with the Head Buyer at the office Christmas party!' This won't get you anywhere at all, and it may put another nail in the coffin of the marriage.

Secondly *don't*, if you can avoid it, react to your partner's infidelity by refusing point blank to make love ever again. It's quite natural to want to refuse to make love with someone who's just let you down. On the other hand you have to remember that love (*including* physical love) is exactly what's needed to 're-cement' your marriage.

Refusing to have sex after things have calmed down might just drive your spouse away for good. Remember that you may well now have competition from 'the other woman' or 'the other man' (in a few cases, from both!).

You need to fight this with all the weapons at your command if you want to retain your spouse. And those include your sexual weapons . . .

Good luck – and I hope you keep your relationship together.

INTERCOURSE

Intercourse – Difficulties In

Sexual problems are extremely common, and it is quite obvious that the physical side of many marriages is unsatisfactory to one partner or both. The situation does seem to be improving, however, and this undoubtedly because people in general are today far less ignorant about love-making than they were 20 or even 10 years ago.

Where a husband and wife have difficulties with intercourse, the best thing is if they both sit down and read a good marriage manual, which can be obtained from places like the Family Planning Association (phone number below) or 'Relate' the National Marriage Guidance Council (01-580 1087). Do choose a recent one, however – many of the books which were written a few years back contain all sorts of dangerous myths and misleading information!

A small (but slowly increasing) number of doctors are now undertaking training in the treatment of sexual problems. If your own doctor can't help you, ask him to refer you to someone who can. If in difficulty, ring the Family Planning Information Service on 01-636 7866.

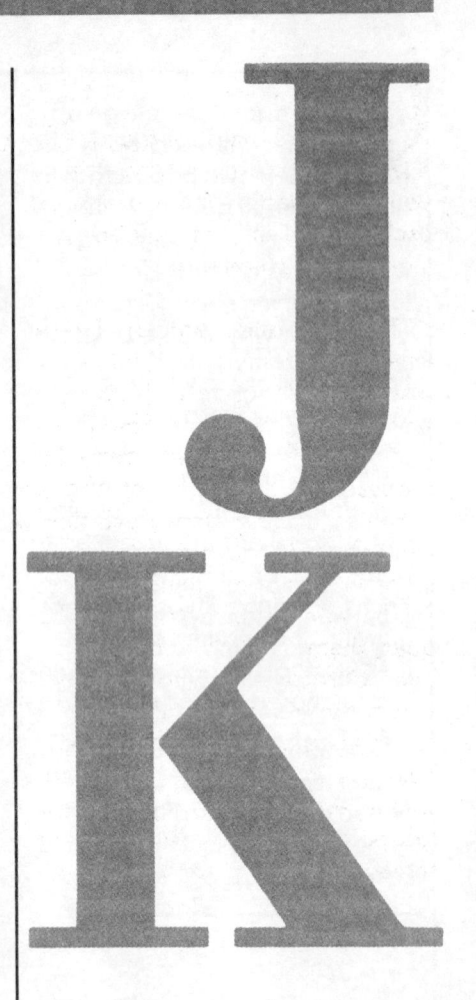

JEALOUSY • KISSING

Q We are a husband and wife in the West Country, writing you a joint letter about a serious problem which has soured our marriage. It is jealousy.

(The husband writes:) Every time I go out, my wife is intensely suspicious about how I feel towards other women. She fears that I will become sexually aroused at the sight of them, becomes acutely depressed and can't sleep. In fact, I don't chat up other women or anything like that.

(The wife writes:) Wherever he goes, there's bound to be at least one attractive woman, about whom he might have thoughts. I see this as mental unfaithfulness. It has got to the stage now that whenever he returns home I have to ask if he has been attracted to someone else.

A Your marriage is heading for disaster unless you do something about it. The most encouraging thing is you've written me a JOINT letter – which does suggest that both of you want to work your way to a solution.

All normal people feel some degree of jealousy over the person they love. (Indeed, when jealousy vanishes, that's often an indication that love has gone.) But in this case, the jealousy has really reached the stage of an obsessional neurosis. In other words, you're now ill. To save your health and your marriage, ask your GP to refer you for psychotherapy immediately.

Having read your husband's contribution to your anguished joint letter, I'm sure he loves you and will help and support you. Good luck to you both.

Q Recently, I was very surprised to find that I was willing to go to bed with a guy and have intercourse, but then discovered that I was really a bit repelled by the idea of having him kiss me. Do you think I am abnormal?

A Nope. For a lot of women, a kiss seems to be more intimate than sexual intercourse.

I'd guess that you weren't very interested in this bloke, this is probably a good indication that you shouldn't waste your time going to bed with him again.

LESBIANISM

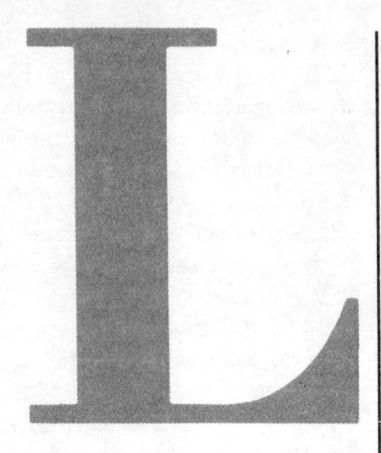

Q My wife and I were engaged in love play the other night when she admitted to me that when she was at university, she'd had a lesbian relationship with a woman who is now one of our best friends. This relevation turned me on at the time, but I'm a bit worried. Do you think my wife might be basically homosexual?

A I really doubt if your missus will turn out to be one of what are sometimes called 'Les Girls'. You see, it is fantastically common in young women to have brief physical relationships with each other, particularly when they're lonely and away from home. When you consider how readily younger women snuggle up to one another and how quite cheerfully they share beds (in a way that would be anathema to most of us chaps!), it's scarcely surprising that they sometimes 'slide over the border' into sexual contact.

As a matter of fact, the amazing Dr Kinsey found that no less than 30% of young college girls had had a physical relationship with another woman. Many of them were probably homesick and need of a cuddle, like your wife perhaps.

To give you a f'rinstance of how common this kind of thing is, even one of Britain's best-known agony

LESBIANISM • LIVING TOGETHER

columnists is perfectly open about having had two youthful homosexual relationships. (And in case anybody's wondering – no, it *isn't* me!).

Q I wonder if you can answer a very difficult question for me?
Why is my husband admitting that he occasionally gets turned on by the idea of lesbianism?

A Can't tell you for certain, but there's no doubt that – bizarrely enough – vast numbers of gents seem to be intrigued by the idea of women caressing each other.
Studies of men's secret fantasies have shown this quite clearly. Furthermore, I am told that both orgies and live 'sex shows' usually feature girl-to-girl lovemaking in an attempt to excite the male audience.
This is really all a bit baffling, isn't it? After all, you don't find women going around proclaiming to be turned on by the idea of guys going in for homosexual lovemaking. (At least, I don't think so anyway.)

Q I am a widow, and after many years of lusty heterosexual life with my late husband. I am amazed to find that I've fallen into an occasional warm lesbian relationship with a dear friend. Is this illegal?

A No ma'am. Oddly enough, lesbian love-making (unlike male homosexual activity) has never been illegal in Britain. It's claimed that this is because of the fact that when the appropriate law was due to be passed in the 19th century, no one had the nerve to explain it to Queen Victoria.

Q I was very upset to learn that my daughter – age 21 – is regularly sleeping with her boyfriend at the weekends. Is there any way I can stop them?

A I fear not, ma'am. I understand how you feel – but life has changed, and the fact is that most young adult women go to bed with their boyfriends these days.
Indeed, a recent survey showed that over a third of under-25s do lead a decidedly more promiscuous life than that – with three or more partners a year. Be grateful that your daughter isn't apparently one of this group, but just has one steady (and, I hope, loving) male friend.

49

LIVING TOGETHER

Living Together

One of the amazing changes of recent years has been the vast increase in the habit of living together. Twenty years ago, you couldn't publicly admit that you were living together: yet nowadays, every other pop star seems to have a 'live-in-lover' – and a very high proportion of young adults are doing the same thing.

In some instances there is a definite case for living together. When I survey the shattered marriages of people who only managed to make it through the first three or four months of matrimony (and then found out they couldn't *stand* one another!), I seriously wonder why they didn't avoid all the trouble and legal complications by living together on a trial basis first.

I note that there is one world-famous female media pundit whose views on marriage are avidly quoted in newspapers and TV. *Her* only marriage lasted three weeks! Why couldn't she just have moved in with the man for a month or two, discovered they were incompatible, and saved the vicar all that trouble for nothing?

Also, there is a widespread feeling today that living together is at least 'stable' and therefore preferable to the promiscuity which so many young adults adopt. On the other hand, there are difficulties and dangers in the 'living-together' relationship. They can be summed up briefly like this:

parents and relatives may still be very upset

you need to be very clear about what happens if somebody gets pregnant – which they frequently do. (If it happens, *don't* rush into matrimony just to 'give the baby a name' – a hurried marriage is *never* a good idea.)

sordid and commercial though it sounds, you've also got to be very clear about what your *financial* arrangements are going to be – regrettably, many live-in couples run into all sorts of bitter financial disputes when they break up. It's a pretty awful business when two former lovers meet up in court to fight over who gets half the house or – in the USA – who pays 'palimony'.

So, think twice before you accept that tempting invitation to 'move in with me, darling!' You could be letting yourself in for a lot of happiness – or for a lot of trouble.

LOVE PLAY

Q My live-in boyfriend is a great guy and a wonderful lover. But he seems to have one problem that I'm too embarrassed to ask him about.

Every time he goes for a pee in the night, he misses the toilet. As a result, there is usually a slight puddle for me to clear up.

Do you think there's anything wrong with him?

A Nope – except he should be clearing up his own 'puddles'.

I must admit that there's a chance that he might have a moderately common anatomical abnormality of the penis (present in about one man in 200), which makes it a bit difficult to avoid peeing on the floor.

But another explanation is much likelier.

When a bloke has been sexually excited, his 'love juices' (as us doctors call them) tend to create a slight blockage in the urinary pipe for a little while.

This makes it very difficult for the gent to 'aim straight' when he next visits the loo. If you ask your boyfriend, I think he'll confirm that this the cause of the damp patch.

Q I was engaging in some very enthusiastic love play with my husband last week when he suddenly said to me, 'Ouch! Don't twist so hard, or you'll break it.'

This quite alarmed me! Is it really possible for a woman to break a man's penis, in the same way that one can break a wrist or an arm?

A Yes, ma'am – this is a risk that all energetic ladies should know about.

Although your husband's penis doesn't have a bone in it (at least not unless he's a badger or something), it does become almost as stiff as bone when he's excited. This is because it's absolutely packed to bursting point with blood.

The blood is contained in three cylinders (each about the size of a panatella cigar) which run the length of his 'John Thomas'.

If you unwisely grasp his erect organ and twist it violently to one side, you can cause an extremely painful fracture of one or more of these cylinders.

This is a genuine surgical emergency if it occurs, and the unfortunate victim has to be taken to hospital. Usually, his penis is then packed in ice – and he may well

LOVE PLAY

have to be taken to theatre to have the blood clot removed from inside it. This is not a lot of fun.

So ladies – whatever you do to your gents in bed, PLEASE eschew all forms of violent twisting manipulation!

However, bear in mind that the secret information which I have imparted to you today can be used as a defence against rapists.

If you are ever attacked by a naked man with an erect penis, simply grasp it as firmly as you can – and forcibly rearrange it from 12 o'clock to six o'clock – and then run like hell.

Q My fiancée has just started using a peppermint 'body lotion' during lovemaking. When it gets into her vagina, it gives us both quite an exciting sensation. But is it safe to use it like this?

A It's quite well-known that peppermint-flavoured lotions do give both partners an agreeable tingle.

However, introducing chemicals and flavourings into the vagina can cause a sensitivity reaction, in which the delicate tissues (yours too) become sore and red. So I reckon that your fiancée should be a little wary about what she puts into her vagina. Come to think of it, that's not a bad maxim for all women everywhere...

Q What worries me is this: since so many men have slightly dirty or scruffy fingernails, couldn't vaginal love play lead to infection?

A Yup – you're right. Digital stimulation of the inside of the vagina is the second commonest form of male-female love play. It is most frequently done with the middle finger.

Now simple inspection of a series of men's hands will quickly demonstrate that not all of their fingernails are 100% clean. (Indeed, at the end of a long working day, this would be bacteriologically impossible.)

So transfer of germs to the vagina does happen – and it's possible that those germs might lead to a vaginal discharge. However, the types of germs found on the fingers aren't usually the same ones which cause a discharge (which is good news).

On the other hand (so to speak) there could also be an association between dirty finger nails and cancer of the cervix. You see, I've been pointing out for years that male manual occupations are linked with a higher risk of

LOVE PLAY

cervical cancer in the female partner.

This is possibly because men who do manual work are more likely to bring home dirt in their fingernails.

So the moral is fairly clear. I don't want to stop anybody's bedtime fun – or to deprive women of a very useful source of sexual fulfilment – but gentlemen readers: do please make sure that anything you put inside a woman is clean! (And I do mean *anything* . . .).

Why Love play?

Yes, why have love play? What's the point of it all?

Quite a few bewildered people (mostly of the male persuasion) ask that question. They can't quite see why sex needs to be more than a question of a man putting his penis inside a woman and thrusting away like mad – just like they do in the men's magazines.

But in the real world, things aren't like that at all! For a start, one thing that every young lad needs to know is that most women will not have a climax unless they are given a little love play – certainly before intercourse, perhaps during it, and possibly afterwards too.

Strange as it may seem, this comes as shattering news to many males. But it's true. The majority of women don't usually reach a climax during intercourse itself – only during love play. So for them, no love play usually means no climax (and, almost certainly, no *multiple* climaxes). Furthermore, every man needs to know that nearly all women find intercourse uncomfortable or even downright painful *if there hasn't been preliminary love play*.

Why? Firstly because love play makes the woman's vagina start secreting those famous 'love juices' which are so absolutely vital to lubricate the process of intercourse. Without them, the vagina would be so dry that intercourse would be very unpleasant indeed for the woman (and not a lot of fun for most men).

Secondly, preliminary love play makes the vaginal muscles — which guard the opening of the vagina — open up in preparation to receive the penis. If a man tries to enter before that initial opening up process is completed, the woman will feel discomfort and even pain. And in the case of some couples, he won't be able to get in at all – this

LOVE PLAY

is a common cause of non-consummation of a marriage!

Thirdly, love play makes the woman's vagina lengthen as she gets more sexually excited – so that there is much more room inside.

But, dear female readers: you aren't the only ones who need love play. Your partner will benefit greatly from it too.

Why? Well, once again let's look at the purely mechanical aspect of sex for a moment. Vast numbers of men have difficulties and worries over their erections. 'Will I be able to get it hard?'...'Will it *stay* hard?...'Will it collapse on me?'

That's one reason why so many of them do stupid things like leap inside a woman the moment they've achieved an erection – they're terrified it might collapse!

But if man's in bed with a woman who is skilled at love play, he need have no anxieties whatever. For with deft fingers and lips, she will assuredly bring him to an erection – perhaps many times in an evening, depending how matters develop.

Indeed, I'm convinced that a woman who is really adept at love play could cure most cases of impotence single-handed (so to speak). Would that there were more such women around!

Actually, even the most active and 'virile' of males who has no doubts or anxieties about his 'performance' will nonetheless benefit from being on the receiving end of skilled love play techniques. This is partly because love play plays such an important role in romance but the other point to make about love play is this. *It's so very nice!*

Romance and Love Play

One of the main reasons that love play is so good is that is awfully romantic! Yes, romantic. Love play is of course the natural progression of, say, a candlelit dinner, with soft lights, sweet music and the gentle touch of the hands across the dining table. Without love play, there can be no romance.

Consider the sort of awful situations in which there is a complete *absence* of love play, and you will see that they represent the exact opposite of romance. Here are a few such situations:

a man going with a prostitute for a five-minute encounter

a man coming home drunk and forcing himself on his wife

a woman being raped

LOVE PLAY

In all of these unpleasant situations, the contact between man and woman is basic, squalid and brutish. There's no romance – and, of course, there's no love play.

How very different when two people love each other and want to make each other happy! Right from the start, they do everything they can to 'pleasure' one another – and to make each other feel good and warm and wanted. In short, they use love play – which is an essential ingredient of any romantic relationship between a man and a woman.

General Caressing

How does love play begin? Well, as you can see from the title of this section, it usually begins with General Caressing. And a fine old soldier he was too...

I use the word 'general' because it is very important that the man – in particular – should always take care to avoid starting with any kind of *direct* approach to the woman's genitals.

Many males don't realize that most females are very definitely turned off by sudden, premature, unsubtle approaches to the vaginal region. Some men hold the touching belief that if you make a quick lunge towards a woman's vagina, she will promptly melt into your arms – but that is, of course, nonsense.

No: what nearly all women prefer is an indirect (and – yes! – romantic) approach in which the man:

says nice things and tells her he loves her

strokes her hair

holds her hand

strokes her shoulders

strokes her arms

strokes her back

All of these actions, you'll notice, are pleasant and arousing – but sexually non-demanding. If a man does them to a woman, she can enjoy them without feeling pressurized. (This was really one of the great discoveries that the old firm of Masters and Johnson made in their researches at their sex clinic in St Louis, Missouri: they found that non-sexual caressing was a great way of building up somebody's confidence and making them feel relaxed and happy.

From this stage, the experienced lover will move on to rather more specifically sexual caresses – but, if he's wise, without yet

LOVE PLAY

making a direct approach to the woman's vagina.

For example, he can:

caress her buttocks

stroke her legs

fondle her breasts

and, of course, kiss these parts of her body too.

Research with the amazing vaginal probe at London's Institute of Psychiatry shows very clearly that while this sort of pleasant caressing is going on, a woman's vagina does start preparing itself for love-making as she becomes more and more aroused.

Much the same principles of gradually increasing stimulation apply if you are a woman caressing your man. However, I have to admit that most men do prefer a rather more direct approach than is favoured by most women. So very few males will complain if a female fairly rapidly starts transferring her attention to his penis. Now read on . . .

Love play with the Fingers

So let's now move on to actual love-play with the fingers – what many people call 'petting'. A lot of people get very embarrassed about this subject, and think that there is something terribly 'rude' about using your fingers to give your loved one sexual pleasure. But in actual fact, it's very hard to see how a couple could have a really good and satisfying sexual relationship if they didn't go in for 'finger-play'. Certainly, very few women would reach orgasm without it. (And still fewer would reach multiple orgasms.)

However, love-play with the fingers is *not* an instinctive thing: you have to know what to do. If you do *not* know what to do, you will hurt your partner!

This is actually very common – especially among newly-weds. The couple leap into bed and, before very long, she makes a lunge for his penis and gives it a rather violent tweak. Result: he doubles up in temporary agony!

More seriously, a man can do a woman quite a lot of harm with clumsy, unskilled attempts at finger petting. What often happens is that he cuts her – externally or internally – with his fingernails. This can cause pain, and quite a lot of bleeding. And, most importantly, the pain may put her off sex for a very long time – and indeed help to cause the common sex difficulty called 'vaginismus'. So, when using finger-play:

be sure your nails aren't jagged

be gentle

if necessary, use a lubricant

make sure you know what you're doing – and

practise!

Now, what exactly do you do! Let us look first at the nice things a man can do for a woman – and then at the equally nice things she can do to him.

Things Men Can Do for Women

OK, so you're going to use your fingertips to give your partner pleasure. Begin by *gently* brushing your fingertips past the opening of her vagina. *Don't* rush things, and don't do anything silly like trying to ram a finger straight in immediately.

Instead, lovingly stroke the outside of her vagina. If you've wooed her carefully, lovingly and romantically, you'll find that she's already beginning to become moist with love juices.

Next, use the pads of your fingers to caress the area of her clitoris. Rub gently on either side of it – or, if she prefers it, rub directly on it (though not all women like this). *Ask her what she likes*. There's no point in lying there doing something that simply doesn't turn her on!

If things are very dry round her clitoris, it may be worthwhile scooping up a little of her love juice on your fingertips. But if there's not much of it around, then there is no reason why you shouldn't lick your fingertips.

Alternatively, some couples use a lubricant, such as baby oil – or one of the lubricants sold in sex shops.

Learning how to stimulate a woman's clitoris properly is one of the great loving arts, which every man should master – though remarkably few do. If in doubt, remember: keep it gentle, but *fast*. And do what she likes – not what *you* think is best!

Once she is really moist, you may well wish to move on to the next stage of finger-play, which is slipping a finger *inside* her vagina. That is a very good preparation for intercourse; if more bridegrooms knew how to do it, there'd be fewer unconsummated marriages.

You can use any of your fingers, but the middle one is usually the most effective. Slide it in gently.

Then move it gently but rapidly

LOVE PLAY

in and out. Do *not* make the movements too vigorous, or you may catch her delicate tissues with your fingernail. If you follow this finger technique properly, you'll find that your thumb or forefinger will, at the same time rub gently against the region of her clitoris – so giving her added stimulation.

I'm not exaggerating when I say that really *mastering* this technique may take you years. Yet mastering it will pay rich dividends, in terms of the pleasure and satisfaction you'll give to your loved one.

But once you are reasonably adept at the 'middle finger method', then you can try some of the following:

put your thumb inside instead, and gently rotate it

put your middle *and* index fingers in, and use the pads of the two fingertips gently to stimulate her G-spot

use your index finger to stimulate the sensitive *sides* of her vagina

use a finger pad to stimulate the back wall of her vagina (though not all women like this, so be guided by what the lady tells you)

use the tips of two fingers to stimulate her cervix gently

At all times, be gentle and sensitive. Take your lead from the speed and intensity of her breathing, from any little moans of pleasure she makes – and, above all, from what she asks you to do!

Things Women Can Do for Men

Now what can a woman do with her fingers to please a man?

Well, we men don't have as many (or as interesting) sex organs as you do. But we do have several areas which are very sensitive to soft female fingertips.

First of all, you can stroke your partner's nipples – most men like this. You will find that his nipple gets a little erection, though not on the same scale as yours.

Next, you can stroke his testicles. This will not bring a man to a climax, but it's an agreeable and sometimes rather comforting sensation for him.

And finally, of course, there's his penis. There are various ways of stimulating this with your fingers. In practice, you need to find out what the man you love likes having done to his organ.

So for heaven's sake, ask him! Half the mix-ups and confusions in people's beds are caused by the fact that so many couples are

LOVE PLAY

too embarrassed to speak while they're trying to get each other excited.

It's not generally known that you may well find it easier to do this sort of love-play if you actually anoint his penis with a little baby oil, or other bland lubricant. I gather that some men prefer talcum powder.

You may also find it helpful to hold his testicles with your other hand while you are gently rubbing his penis. Girls in massage parlours (who, I assume, probably know more about this than most people) have a technique in which they increase pleasurable tension in the penis by holding the testicles downwards with one hand while they rub the male organ with the other.

All these finger techniques are useful in adding fun and fulfilment to a loving relationship. Don't worry – as some women do – that you will damage your partner's penis by handling it. (Remember, you're far more likely to damage his ego by *not* handling it.)

However, in a vigorous session of love play, you should take care not to do two things when it's erect:

don't twist it violently to one side – this is an occasional cause of quite serious injury (it's also quite a good thing to do to a would-be rapist!)

don't 'twang' it back violently towards his feet – when it's erect, it's *not* meant to go that way.

Love play with the Lips and Tongue

Naturally, the mouth plays a very important part in love play. Kissing your partner all over is immensely agreeable – as is being kissed all over in return.

When you are doing this, you can of course combine caressing with your tongue. And don't forget those little nibbles and 'love-bites', which most people like being on the receiving end of.

But... it's best not to go in for love-bites around the sexual parts of the body, where they may cause damage and excessive pain.

What about love-biting the breasts? Some women like this, others don't – and may even be frightened by it. It's probably best not to love-bite the nipples (which are very sensitive in both sexes) but just to confine yourself to gentle sucking.

Now to the controversial subject of kissing the 'naughty bits'. I don't know why people

LOVE PLAY

still get so het up about this subject, but a lot of them are offended by it, even today.

In fact, kissing someone in their most intimate part is the most natural and delightful way of showing your love – and of giving him or her great pleasure. It's certainly not to everybody's taste, but research does indicate that the majority of younger couples now go in for it.

Mouth-play for a Man to Use on a Woman

So how can a man pleasure the woman he loves by using his lips and tongue? It's really quite simple. If you're a man who isn't used to this sort of thing, then just begin by giving long, lingering kisses to the upper part of your partner's pubic hair.

From there, you can move down and gently kiss the region of her clitoris. This gives most women tremendous pleasure and satisfaction – and it's a very useful way of helping the woman who has difficulty in reaching a climax.

Next you can gently titillate her clitoris with the tip of your tongue. This isn't easy to begin with, but after a little practice you'll find it tremendously effective in pleasing her.

Finally, there's a technique which gives many women great pleasure, but which not all men are keen on trying. It involves actually putting the tongue inside her vagina.

It's certainly well worth having a go at, though it's like oysters – a bit of an acquired taste! All you do is gently insert your tongue into your partner's vagina, and gently move it in and out. This is very effective – though if the lady gets very enthusiastic, you may find it a trifle difficult to draw breath!

Mouth-play for a Woman to Use on a Man

Now, what nice things can a woman do for her partner with her mouth? Basically it's just a question of using your lips and tongue to give him pleasure. You can, if you wish, take one of his testicles in your mouth – be very gentle since they are rather sensitive!

You can also kiss the area of skin just *behind* his testicles – an area which is very sexually receptive in most males.

But the thing which men appreciate most is direct stimulation of the penis. You can do this in three ways:

simply kissing it (a nice, loving thing to do)

LOVE PLAY

licking it with your tongue (this is very sexually stimulating – and a great help to the man who has difficulty getting an erection)

putting it in your mouth and sucking (be careful not to give him a painful jab with your teeth!)

Once again, oral love-play techniques on the penis (termed 'fellatio') aren't to *everybody's* taste. But research shows that a very high proportion of couples do now enjoy it.

Incidentally, you'll find that these oral love play techniques on your partner are often best performed while he's doing much the same thing to you. This involves taking up the famous '69' or '*soixante-neuf*' position, in which the couple's bodies roughly resemble the figure '69' on the bed.

Putting Things in the Vagina

Be very cautious about putting anything in the vagina except what nature intended for it! Unfortunately, some of those frightful and tacky men's magazines at the cheaper end of the market have given a lot of young males the notion that it's a good idea to play silly games with cucumbers, bananas and whatnot. This no way to get your vitamin C!

Seriously, foreign bodies might possibly carry infection. *Hard* foreign bodies can damage the vagina – I have certainly encountered one case in which terrible damage was done to a woman because her husband was stupid enough to put a wooden rod inside.

And most hospital casualty officers are familiar with those incredible cases in which a woman arrives in an ambulance with a bottle or a jar jammed inside her. It's all right to put a clean vibrator in the vagina if you want to do so, but no other objects.

Incidentally, words fail me at the idea given world-wide prominence in Shirley Conran's novel *Lace* – that a man can give a woman pleasure by putting a *goldfish* inside her vagina. If I heard of anybody doing such a stupid thing, I'd report them to the RSPCA (and that isn't a joke!)

Rectal Love Play or 'Bottom-play'

This seems to be almost universal among sophisticated couples these days (partly as a result of the influence of Marlon Brando's film *Last Tango in Paris*). I suppose it's not altogether surprising, since nature for some

LOVE PLAY

reason has equipped the bottom with a lot of sexually excitable nerve endings.

Rather astonishingly, there's no doubt that many women can reach a climax simply through having the rectal opening gently stimulated with a fingertip. This activity is called *postillionage*.

Also, as readers of Harold Robbins novels will know, it's quite easy for a woman to slip a well-lubricated finger up a man's bottom and massage his prostate gland. This definitely helps some men get aroused, and gives an intense and rather unusual climax.

But... what the films and novels don't make clear is that the back passage is, of course, a germ-laden area of the body. To be blunt, a finger placed there will come away with germs on it. As you probably know there's now not the slightest doubt that the germ of AIDS can be transmitted by the rectal activities of homosexual blokes.

I'm not suggesting that tickling your loved one's backside will give you AIDS. But if you decide to go in for this sort of thing, then at the very least you ought to wash your hand afterwards. On no account put it near her/his genitals (or your own) till this has been done.

Incidentally, bottom-play without a lubricant is likely to be *very* uncomfortable, and may cause bleeding. This is why sales of butter are alleged to have gone up so dramatically after the aforementioned Marlon Brando film.

Using Drugs to Heighten Love play

This is widespread – and absolutely mad. I cannot over-emphasize the fact that drugs like heroin, cocaine and the various substances that people 'sniff' are likely to take away your sex drive, ruin your health, and very possibly kill you.

Some experts appear to think that *small* amounts of alcohol and 'pot' (which is, of course, illegal in most countries) can safely be used to relax people and so make love play more agreeable. However, any doctor will tell you that *larger* amounts of alcohol have a serious adverse effect on people's love-lives – hence the well-known euphemism for impotence: 'brewer's droop'.

To sum up, don't spoil your love play with drugs. They aren't a passport to instant happiness – in fact, they're more likely to be a passport to the grave.

MAKING LOVE

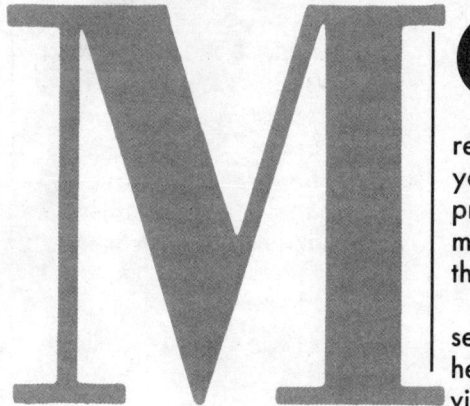

Q I am a married woman of 40, and my husband is 50. I recently had a short affair with a young man of 20, and was surprised to find that he was able to make love to me much more often than my husband is.

My husband is only able to have sex once a night. Is there anything he could take to make him more virile?

A No, ma'am. And if your husband is making love once a night at 50, he's doing very well. The average man of 50 does it less than twice a week.

And it's normal for a man of 20 to be able to make love to you much more often than a bloke of 50 can. After all, 20 goes into 40 more often than 50 does...

Q I am much more interested in sex than my husband, so I have to persuade him (verbally and manually) to make love as often as I want to. My worry is this: could I do him any harm by over-stimulating him?

A No – it's impossible to harm any man or woman by 'over-stimulating' them. The worst that will

MAKING LOVE • MARRIAGE

happen is that he may get a trifle tired.

Q My husband (aged 35) used to be a very enthusiastic lover, but nowadays he doesn't seem to be interested in making love to me for a second time during an evening. Do you think he's losing his virility?

A Like many people, you're expecting too much orgasmically of your partner! Many men can only manage it once in an evening. And at 35, the average male has about two orgasms per week. So let the poor bloke rest if he wants to.

Q My husband – age 40 – can only make love once in an evening. Previous lovers of mine could do it twice. Is he OK?

A Perfectly OK, ma'am. Unfortunately, many women do tend to overestimate the ability of us chaps to achieve multiple climaxes.
In fact, the ability to make love more than once in an evening depends largely on age.
Research indicates that the percentage of men who regularly (as opposed to occasionally) 'come' more than once in a night is roughly as follows:

Under 16	20%
16–20	15%
21–30	9%
31–40	6%
41–50	2.5%
51–60	3.5%

Q I had a hysterectomy four months ago, but no one has said anything about making love to my husband again. I feel I am being unfair to him, and I also want to make love. How soon can we?

A I find it incredible that no one at the hospital had the sense to tell you this. Following most hysterectomies, it's possible to start making love (with care) about six weeks after the op, but always ask your surgeon.

Q I am a young Asian woman, and I became pregnant as a result of rape. I had a termination, and the man then blackmailed me into having sex with him again. This led to another termination of pregnancy. But I am now free of this man's influence.

MARRIAGE

The problem is that my parents have now arranged a marriage for me. Would my bridegroom-to-be be able to tell that I have had two abortions?

A. No, he wouldn't. I'm dreadfully sorry to read your appalling story. Quite frankly, it makes my fists itch to thump the bloke who raped and blackmailed you. I think that before you embark on matrimony, you desperately need some personal advice and counselling – eg from the *Brook Advisory Centres For Young People*. Ring their HQ on 01-580 2991. Good luck.

Q. I have just got married, and the thing I find most embarrassing about living with a man for the first time is that he is able to hear me pee when I visit the loo, which has a very thin door! How can I cope with this?

A. Well ma'am, in the *short* term, you could get a thicker loo door – or just turn the taps on while you're spending a penny. But in the long term, this is one of the things that couples simply have to adjust to. It may take some years before you feel equable about your man overhearing the tinkling noises produced by your bodily functions.

Marriage

Obviously, this book can't be a complete and infallible treatise on marriage. But from the experience of watching a large number of savable marriages break up – mainly because one or both parties persisted in behaving in a way that was silly, immature and selfish – I would suggest these few almost laughably simple ground rules:

when you have problems, *talk* to your partner: 'bottling it up' is likely to lead to disaster

try every day to *praise* your partner – not to criticize him or her

if things are going wrong sexually, *seek professional help* before matters get any worse

try not to commit adultery – it's awfully common, but the troubles it can bring are enormous

if you *do* commit adultery, keep quiet about it; if you must unburden some guilt, find a good friend, doctor, priest or counsellor to talk to, but don't shift the unhappiness onto your poor old spouse

if you suspect or find out that your partner has had an affair,

MARRIAGE

> try not to regard it as the end of the marriage
>
> don't seek answers to marriage problems in drink or drugs – a very high proportion of divorces are related to alcohol abuse
>
> don't involve your children in difficulties between you and your spouse – and never try to 'recruit' them onto your side
>
> if the going's get rough, always go and see a trained marriage guidance counsellor ('Relate' is the new name for the Marriage Guidance Council)
>
> try to ensure that your partner is sexually happy: an awful lot of men and women pay no real attention to their spouses' sexual needs – and then wonder why the said spouse goes off with somebody else.
>
> If all that advice sounds a bit trite, I can tell you that I have known quite a few couples who've managed to save their marriages by deciding to stick to rules like these, after a period in which they had been very close to breaking up.

Q My boyfriend has a great body, and is truly fantastic in bed. He would like us to get married. But the big problem is this. Don't think me snobbish, but he comes from a much lower social class than me, and it's not just that, my Mum thinks he's 'awfully rough', and quite unsuitable, darling', the real point is that I am a university graduate, and he is a labourer, and the difference in our IQs must be 40 or 50 points.

A I take it you're telling me that yours is bigger than his?

Seriously, I don't think the difference in your 'social standing' is all that important these days. After all, I've known doctors marry lorry-drivers.

But a 40 or 50-point difference in IQ is another matter. Be warned. This bloke may be a great lover, but if his IQ is 90 and yours is 135, you're not going to have a lot to talk about. That's a classic case of a Radio 3 woman marrying a Radio 1 man.

Q I have had to have a mastectomy. I'm 23, about to be married, and my fiancé honestly accepts me as I am, which is marvellous.

But I cannot think of my body as

attractive, and I feel that other people would be shocked if they know how I looked without clothes.

A I bet you look very nice without clothes – and I'm sure that your fiancé will demonstrate (through his physical love) just how attractive you really are.

Meantime, you need help in building up your confidence, and in dealing with the practical difficulties of having lost a breast. Please contact the splendid *Mastectomy Association*, at 26 Harrison Street, London, WC1H 8JG.

Q Something very upsetting happened to me recently. First, I should explain that I was widowed at an early age, and have brought up my daughter on my own. She is now a teenager.

I don't have any boyfriends, but I do have sexual feelings, which for a long time I have relieved by masturbation.

A few months ago, I was lying on my bed, relieving my sexual tensions in this way. To my embarrassment, my daugher walked in.

She was terribly shocked. I could not reason with her, and in fact the whole thing has caused a dreadful rift between us. She has

Masturbation

A surprising number of women still think that there's something wrong or shameful about masturbation – and a few still believe that it has harmful effects, like damaging your eyesight!

But I think most people are now aware that masturbation is completely harmless. Survey after survey has shown that the majority of women have masturbated at some time.

Indeed, this widespread knowledge has itself led to a new source of confusion. There are now quite a few women who think they're 'abnormal' because they don't masturbate! Nothing could be further from the truth. Though the sex surveys do show that the vast majority of adult females have masturbated at some time or other, the fact is that a very substantial number *haven't*. And even among those women who *have* gone in for it, there are many for whom it's just a very intermittent sort of pleasure – often amounting to little more than a comforting stroke through the nightdress on a cold winter's evening.

So medically speaking, the point about masturbation is that it's entirely up to you. Whether you do it or not, you're definitely

MASTURBATION

not 'abnormal'. It's true that many sex therapists do now believe that masturbation is a help to a lot of women: as a reliever of tension; as an aid when there's difficulty in reaching orgasm; and even in relieving a period pain. But no one is obliged to do it!

However, just a few words of warning: women (like men) sometimes do rather silly things when masturbating. For instance, a doctor friend of mine treated a young woman who'd done appreciable harm to her vagina by putting an electric toothbrush inside it. Similarly, I've recently had several letters from doctors about patients who have caused injuries to their clitorises by over-violent manipulation with various objects. And there are also occasional cases of women who very unwisely try to masturbate by pushing things like hairgrips in and out of the urinary pipe. This is madness – there's a high risk that the object will vanish up into the bladder!

So if you want to masturbate (and for many women – especially single, divorced or widowed women – it's undoubtedly a pleasant and soothing experience) it's best to stick to gentle rubbing alongside the clitoris, using either a finger or a vibrator, as you prefer!

---

scarcely spoken to me since then, and is obviously quite disgusted by what she saw.

AThis is awfully sad. I'm afraid it's a fact that one generation finds it hard to come to terms with another generation's sexuality – and your poor daughter simply cannot adjust to the idea that you (her Mum) are a sexual being with normal sexual urges.

To begin with, the most important thing you can do is show her all the love and tenderness you can – no matter how she rejects you. If you get cross with her (which would be very understandable), it'll only confirm her bitter opinion of you.

Next, if you can get her talking, it's vital that you try and get over to her that you *still* love her Dad and think fondly of him. She probably worships his memory, and feels that you were being 'unfaithful' to him.

It might be worth saying to her that many men would actually *prefer* their widows to go on feeling sexy. In a way, it's a tribute to the warm love-life that they once shared together.

It would be nice if you could persuade your daughter to go

MASTURBATION

along with you to one of the *Brook Advisory Centres for Young People* (HQ phone number *01 580 2991*) to have a chat with one of their counsellors – who would, I think, say the same sort of things that I've said here. Good luck.

Q I have a nagging worry about my lover, who is 26. (I am 39.) We've been together for three years, and have a very active sex life, with no inhibitions.

One night we made love several times, and also enjoyed several other forms of sex play.

But the next morning, he told me that during the night he'd woken up feeling very aroused, and couldn't get back to sleep. So he'd gone into the bathroom and masturbated.

I can't understand why he needs to do this on his own. It's as if he'd done it in a world of his own that I don't seem to be part of.

A I do understand that you must have felt 'excluded' by the fact that he went off alone in the middle of the night and had a climax.

But the truth is that many people do 'touch themselves up' when their partners are asleep.

Your partner is clearly a young virile guy who needs quite a lot of sex. He obviously didn't want to disturb your sleep – after a hectic evening's love-making – and I think you should concentrate on the fact that he was thoughtful enough and considerate enough *not* to wake you up and demand more sex.

Which – let's face it – is what a heck of a lot of more selfish people would have done!

Q I recently married my second husband, who is aged 53. He is rather unwilling to make love in the mornings (which is my favourite time), unless I first stimulate him manually. Is he impotent?

A Not at all, ma'am! Like vintage motor cars, many men above a certain age do need to be started by hand – especially on these chilly morns. *Do* warm your hands first, won't you?

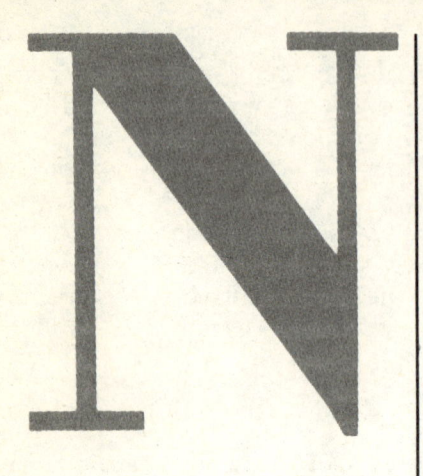

Naughty Underwear

I think it's perfectly reasonable to say that naughty underwear could put a bit of extra fun into a couple's relationship – and perhaps get their love-life going.

The common items are see-through and 'baby-doll' nighties, G-strings, peek-a-boo bras, and open-crotch knickers. For males, there are also *very* abbreviated briefs and 'posing pouches'.

I need hardly say that you don't have to go to a sex shop to get naughty undies. A lot of these items can now be bought quite easily (and possibly considerably cheaper) in high street stores.

Q My fiancé and I were reading your article about lactation when he squeezed his nipple – and out came a little fluid! Why?

A He must have felt a right ...er... wally! Seriously, men do sometimes produce a milky fluid – particularly if their nipples have been stimulated. Some tranquillisers can also make a man secrete a little 'milk'.

THE NIPPLE

Q My husband wants me to put a couple of gold rings through my nipples. Do you think I should agree to this?

A I don't think so – unless it's what *you* want to do.

I reckon that there's been a regrettable increase in all this 'body jewellery' nonsense as a result of the publicity surrounding Sally Beauman's best-selling novel *Destiny* – in which a female character is said to wear a diamond in an unusual and extremely uncomfortable place (a place where it would be a *very* serious hazard for any gent who wanted to make love to her!)

Seriously, 'body piercing' in order to insert jewellery into your delicate places does carry quite a risk of causing infection, bleeding, and pain. I wouldn't have anything to do with it if I were you.

The Nipple

The nipple is one of the most sexually sensitive areas of the body – *in both women and men*. Quite a few women can actually reach a climax just through having their nipples stimulated, although I don't know of any males who experience this.

Most people use the word 'nipple' wrongly – they think it means the *whole* of the pigmented disc in the middle of the breast, but it is, in fact, only the central protuberance; the disc which surrounds it is called the areola. The areola is quite sensitive too, but it does not have as many nerve endings as the nipple. The areola may be pink, brown or black – depending on your general colouring. It can be anything up to 12.5 cm (5 ins) across, and there's no 'normal' size. People are sometimes worried by the little 'blobs' which often run round the areola but these are perfectly normal structures called 'the tubercles of Montgomery'.

The nipple itself contains the openings of the 15–20 milk ducts which are directly connected to one of the most important emotional regions of your brain. That's one reason why both suckling a baby *and* sexual stimulation of the nipple both tend to have a very immediate emotional impact on almost all women.

The Male Nipple

A man's nipple is a sexually excitable organ. That's because it

THE NIPPLE • NUDITY

comes from the same basic tissues which go to form the *female* nipple, and has much the same nerve supply. The only thing that makes the female nipple different is that female hormones have made it grow and develop – and made the breast form around it.

If you give a man female hormones, he too will develop female-looking nipples and breasts.

The fact that the ordinary male's nipple has such a rich nerve supply means that a woman can produce a very good reaction in her partner by stroking it, kissing it, or teasing it gently with her tongue – in fact, just what most women like men to do to *their* nipples.

Nipple erection

When a woman becomes sexually aroused, the nipple promptly starts to stand out. US sex researchers Johnson and Masters say that it may lengthen by as much as a centimetre. But just before orgasm, the surrounding areola also becomes rather engorged – which is why the nipple appears less prominent at that moment.

Why should the nipple become erect anyway? The only reason I can think of is that it's an undoubted fact that the erect nipple is more sexually attractive.

That's why the female nude is traditionally depicted with erect nipples. Renoir's *blondes baigneuses*, today's pin-ups, and the showgirls of Paris are all part of this tradition. Indeed, in Paris theatres they're supposed to keep a feather in the wings – so that the performers can go on stage in a suitably outstanding condition . . .

Q For some time now, I have been extremely irritated about seeing naked or half-naked females on films, TV and video. My boyfriend doesn't agree with me, but I think that it is unbalanced and unfair to show nude women and not nude men. I feel that if they show one, they ought to show the other – otherwise, it's degrading to women. What is your opinion?

A I'm inclined to agree with you. Quite a lot of women – though certainly not all – do like looking at naked men, and I don't see why their wishes should be frustrated. In fact, I *am* available for ladies' luncheon parties.

OPEN MARRIAGE

Open Marrriage

Quite a few people these days are perfectly agreeable to their partners sleeping with other folk. Where a couple reach such an arrangement with each other, it's called an 'open marriage'.

It all sounds very civilized and sophisticated, but often it *doesn't* work out: maybe one partner gets jealous or even violent, or perhaps one or other party will fall in love with someone they've bedded. And then there are dangers of infection and 'outside' pregnancy.

Furthermore, if you have children, it can be very unsettling for them to observe – as they're almost certain to do – that some nights Mummy sleeps with Bill, or Fred, or Jim, or Pierre, or Helmut...

Rather reluctantly, I have to say that some open (or, at least fairly open) marriages work. An alleged example was that of the late and much-loved Lord Louis Mountbatten and his immensely-admired wife Edwina. But the success of that highly unusual relationship depended on the fact that Mountbatten was almost totally devoid of jealousy, and apparently didn't mind in the least whether his wife actually decided to give herself to their

ORAL SEX • ORGASM

> close friend Prime Minister Nehru or not.
>
> From personal observation of people who have tried to work an open marriage policy, I'd say that very few couples could have achieved that kind of non-jealous harmony. I'd even go further and say that most open marriages are likely to end in open divorce.

Q I am a reader in the Middle East. I do not know much about sex. I would like to know if any health problems could be caused by swallowing sperms.

A Well, ma'am, it's not everybody's cup of tea (so to speak), but plenty of women do it. It's certainly not dangerous to your health – but whether it's against the law in the Middle East, I just wouldn't know.

Q I'm in love with a gorgeous male. The problem is that I get so wet and slippery before we start to make love. There is so little friction that sometimes he can't reach a climax.

Is there anything I could do to control the excessive production of 'love juices?'

A 'Fraid not. But he could use a sheath – preferably a 'ribbed' one – which would give more friction.

Another trick is to put your legs together (i.e. between his) during love-making; this 'squeezes' him very slightly and should help to increase the friction.

In fact, if your relationship settles down, you'll probably find that you no longer have quite such violent outpourings of secretion as soon as he gets near you.

Q My husband shouts so loud while climaxing that I'm afraid he can be heard at the end of the road.

He says he shouts because sex is marvellous – and gets better and better! Is this sort of reaction common in men?

A Not really, ma'am. Women do mostly shriek – or at least squeak – when they reach orgasm. But the majority of blokes just gasp or groan a bit.

Still, I think it's great that your husband is so appreciative of your charms – especially as I understand he's in his 60s!

Orgasm

At the medical journal where I work, we still get a steady flow of letters from a small number of doctors who firmly believe that women do not reach an orgasm.

This is manifestly not true! Female orgasm is a widespread and – it would appear – intensely pleasurable event. Judging by the descriptions which women give ('The moment when all the fuses blow', and so on), it seems to be just as nice for you as male orgasm is for us men.

Studies by the amazing sex researchers Virginia Johnson and Dr William Masters – who carried out some truly exotic lab experiments with intra-vaginal cameras and whatnot – seem to confirm without the slightest doubt that most women do reach a climax, in the sense of a dramatic and delightful discharge in the nervous system, in much the same way as men do.

Indeed, the experiments of Johnson and Masters (please note the careful non-sexist reversal of their names!) taught us more about the physiology of female climaxes than we'd ever known before.

Women have a great advantage over men in that – in theory at least – they're capable of second, third, fourth, or fifth climaxes in quick succession. For most men, that's just a pipe dream (if you'll forgive the phrase).

But don't let's get this business of multiple orgasm out of proportion. Kinsey's statistics indicated that only about one woman in seven went in for these multiple climaxes. I'd say that a few more women have multiple orgasms today, but most are perfectly happy with one orgasm at a time, thank you very much.

Now we have to face the fact that there are also many women who *don't* reach a climax, and who are often very upset about it. About 20% of young married women say that they have not yet experienced an orgasm – though the percentage is far smaller among women of more mature years.

I would like to dispose of the old myth that orgasm is supposed to originate from stimulation of one part of your body only – and that anything else is 'wrong'.

Your nervous system can blow its top as a result of stimulation of your vagina, your clitoris, your G-spot, your buttocks, or your breasts – or indeed your ears, if enough sweet nothings are whispered into them. Whatever turns you on, enjoy it!

ORGASM

Multiple Orgasm

People do get either very excited or very upset about this business of multiple orgasm. When **SHE** published an article about *male* multiple orgasm, it aroused great interest – and also some indignation that the subject should be mentioned at all.

Well, what's the truth about *female* multiple orgasm? Does it happen? If so, how many times can it happen? What proportion of women 's experience it? And does it matter if you don't experience it?

Let me answer that last question first. If you don't have multiple orgasms, it doesn't matter two hoots. It doesn't matter how many times you can 'ring the bell' – what counts is whether you're *happy* with your sex life.

From what I've said, you'll gather that there really is no physiological doubt that multiple organsm does happen in some women. The extraordinary laboratory experiments of Johnson and Masters (not to mention their indefatigable – and improbable – vaginal camera) in the USA have made this quite clear.

So how many climaxes can a woman have? Anecdotal evidence indicates that under the right circumstances, three, four or five orgasms would be quite common.

With the help of a skilled lover, it's certainly quite easy for a very small proportion of women to knock up (say) 15 or 20 climaxes in a single night – though they do tend to feel a bit flaked out next day!

I have heard fantastic tales of the occasional very passionate woman being able to have 100 or even 200 orgasms in an evening, though it's very hard to know whether to place any credence in such claims.

Now to the crunch question. What proportion of women do genuinely experience multiple orgasms?

It' not easy to answer that one. Dr Kinsey's researches on American women back in 1953 suggested that only about one woman in seven could have multiple climaxes.

But that was a long time ago, and women have generally become much less inhibited since then. Ms Shere Hite's recent US sex surveys seem to suggest that a rather higher proportion of women had multiple orgasms. And our recent **SHE** surveys indicate that many British women reach multiple orgasm IF they're adequately stimulated.

ORGASM

Female Orgasm

Let me set out the physiological facts, as discovered by the intrepid team of Masters and Johnson.

What happens at orgasm is this. At the supreme moment of pleasure, most of the muscles of your body go into a quite uncontrollable spasm.

During that period of the orgasm when your eyes are open, your pupils can be seen to be big and dreamy – this is an effect of adrenaline, coursing through your bloodstream.

Your face – could you but see it, dear reader – contorts into an expression which may be like the widest of smiles, but which more commonly is almost like a grimace of pain. But of course, it's not pain that causes it – it's ecstasy (I hope).

Even your toes curl up with pleasure – one of the most reliable signs of orgasm to anyone who happens to be in the regions of a woman's feet at the moment of climax (unusual, I'll admit).

What else? The mouth of your vagina – which has become swollen into a sort of soft collar intended to fit snugly round the base of your man's penis – now starts to contract in a series of highly pleasureable waves.

These waves occur roughly once a second – that is, with much the same frequency as the 'surges' of a man's climax. Several readers have misunderstood what I said about these vaginal contractions, and thought I was claiming they didn't happen. Yes – they do occur: but the point is that a man can't normally feel them (which is why it's so easy for a woman to fake orgasm).

Elsewhere in the book, on the pages headed 'clitoral erection' and 'nipple erection', I have explained the breast changes which take place at orgasm. Another orgasmic change is a curious measles-like rash, which briefly appears in fair-skinned women just as they 'come.'

Finally, there's one other event associated with female orgasm – *le cri*. The characteristic 'climax cry' is evinced by most – though not all – women at the very apogee of the climactic experience.

I'm not kidding when I say that this really is a very useful sound – because it does give a man the best possible indication that his loved one has 'got there'.

It's also a curiously disturbing and erotic sound when you hear it through the thin walls of a hotel bedroom. But that's another story.

ORGASM

Male Orgasm

We've already discussed female orgasm. So let's be even-handed and investigate the same function as it occurs in men. How does your man reach *his* orgasm?

Well, the extraordinary lab experiments of Johnson and Masters in the US have shown that there are quite a few similarities between male and female orgasms. For instance, a bloke has his climax in four basic stages, just as a woman does.

The excitement phase is simply the one in which he has achieved an erection and is getting more and more enthusiastic about you.

The plateau phase is the one in which he remains more or less in control of himself, but could 'fire off' at any time. In successful relationships, this agreeable plateau can, if wished, be prolonged for half an hour or more.

The ejaculation phase is of course very brief, and corresponds to what you experience at the height of your own orgasm. A man's muscular contractions at this stage occur with much the same frequency as those experienced by a woman.

The resolution phase is the rather pleasant 'afterglow' time, during which the man's sex organs return to their normal state.

You'll notice that after the ejaculation phase, there's what the sexperts call a refractory period. This means the time during which a man cannot respond again, no matter what you do to him. Only after the refractory period is over can he have another climax.

In younger men, the refractory period can be quite short – sometimes only a matter of minutes. In older men, however, it may last some days. I have to say that because of the refractory period, multiple orgasm is rare in gents, although there are a few recorded cases. Multiple orgasm in men is entirely dependent on age.

Indeed, the solid and dependable researches of Dr Kinsey indicate that the percentage of blokes who can reach multiple orgasm at various ages is as follows:

Age	Percentage
Under 16	20%
16–20	15%
21–30	9%
31–40	6%
41–50	2.5%
51–60	3.5%

I suppose this goes some way toward explaining why so many women today take younger lovers...

ORGASM

Q I have a very good marriage, but though I can reach a climax easily through petting, I can't do it during actual sex. Am I abnormal?

A Nope. Several studies carried out over the last few years indicate that – contrary to what's generally believed – most women *don't* usually reach an orgasm during intercourse – only during love play. Women who regularly 'ring the bell' during actual intercourse are fortunate, but in a minority.

Q This is a most embarrassing question, but I would like to sort it out before I marry my fiancé.

The trouble is this. When we dance together, he keeps having a climax in his trousers! We've never had sex together, partly because we're both shy. What could he do to avoid it?

A Has he ever considered wearing a kilt?

Seriously, lots of young chaps have had the embarrassing experience of 'coming' in their pants while dancing with a pretty girl. The friction of the trousers and the pressure of the girl's body can combine to have explosive effects when a nervous young man is on a short fuse.

In other words, he may well have the very common male condition called 'premature ejaculation', or 'hair-trigger trouble'. You won't find this out for certain until you try and make love to him.

The important thing now is to talk to him about it, treating the subject with sympathy and humour.

Meanwhile, if you agree not to bother with dances for a while, this would take the pressure off him (in more ways than one).

Q I am a 21-year-old girl from Ireland and am very shy. I had a boyfriend, but he wanted to make love to me. When I said I didn't want to, he went away.

Since then I have been very depressed. And when I go out, everyone stares at me.

Recently I have taken to cuddling up and 'making love' with a teddy bear, and this brings me to a climax. Is that harmful?

A Would that be the teddy bear with the big smile on his face by any chance?

Seriously, what you've been doing with 'Big Ted' is quite harmless – and I'm sure no-one with any

ORGASM

sense would blame you for seeking solace in this way at such a difficult time.

As you say, you're fairly depressed. The feeling that 'everyone is looking at me' is very characteristic of depression.

So I do urge you to go and get some help from your doc now. You also need some 'self-assertiveness' training to help you overcome your shyness.

If there isn't a psychologist in your area who offers this kind of training, write to the *Institute of Behaviour Therapy*, who have self-assertiveness tapes and books, and arrange seminars for shy people. The address is: *38, Queen Anne Street, London W1*.

Q I can climax when my husband pets me, but not when we have intercourse, as a rule. Is there something wrong with me?

A Nope. As I've said several times in this column, one of the great myths about sex is that most women regularly climax during intercourse.

The admirable US statistician Ms Shere Hite has shown in her massive American surveys that this is quite untrue. Most women don't reach an orgasm regularly during actual intercourse, as opposed to love-play.

I once had the very enjoyable experience of having tea at the Ritz with Ms Hite, and she made this point very forcefully, over the cucumber sandwiches. (I was profoundly grateful that she didn't order crumpet.)

Q While I was driving along the M6 to visit my husband in Liverpool, I found that I was stroking myself to pass the time away. There was no danger of me losing control of the car, but I did actually reach a climax. Do you think this was wrong?

A Well, as long as it was only the M6... I do understand that the long stretch before the Sandbach turn-off can be more than trifle tedious. But next time you feel a little bored on the motorway, it may prove a little safer just to turn on the radio (rather than yourself).

Q I am 47 years old, happily married for 23 years, and have never had a climax.

Some years ago, I discovered the vibrator. With the use of it, I have been able to experience feelings that I'd never had before.

ORGASM

My heart races, I perspire and pant, and I have to shout out as my legs and body stiffen.

The feeling that I have is quite fantastic. But though I have been to various doctors and sex therapists. I cannot 'click over' into a climax. Please help.

A Well, ma'am to be quite frank, it sounds to me as though what you're having at the moment *is* an orgasm, by most people's definitions.

I know you feel that there's something *more* which you should be experiencing. But people's climaxes do vary a great deal and to a lot of women, what you describe in your letter would be a climax.

I don't think you should keep 'striving' for more: this is rarely productive where orgasms are concerned. To be honest, I think that you're lucky that you're happily married and that you're experiencing sexual sensations which you yourself describe as 'fantastic'.

Q I am a young lady from Cambridge, and I am made to feel inadequate because my boyfriend says that I do not 'come'.

But I think that I do! However, he says that it is impossible for a woman to reach orgasm without gushing forth fluid at the moment of ecstacy.

A It's your boyfriend who's gushing, dear young lady from Cambridge! He's not a St John's man, is he?

Honestly, he's really got this the wrong way round. It has recently been established that a small proportion of women do seem to produce some sort of fluid at the moment of orgasm. But the vast majority do NOT!

So if you think you're 'coming' at Cambridge, I'm sure you're the one who is right.

Q I am usually on the very brink of a climax when my husband 'comes'. He then falls asleep immediately, leaving me frustrated! Do ALL men make a habit of doing this?

A Many do, dear lady. It's thought that immediately after orgasm, a sedative chemical floods through a man's brain – making him very sleepy, unless he fights against it. And that's why it may be a good 10 minutes or so before a man can lift a finger (if you'll forgive the phrase).

However if you stress to your

ORGASM

husband that you really want him to stay awake and 'finish you off', I'm sure he'll try. The alternative would be to buy a vibrator – you never know, the buzzing might wake him up.

Q In answer to your question about being multi-orgasmic, we can only answer that in this household, we do not know. But we would be very interested to find out.

We are two potentially multi-orgasmic females, and as yet we have not found a skilled lover.

If you would like to send one round, we would be willing to try him out, in the aid of scientific research – and we will forward the results of the experiment on to you.

A Would male readers kindly note that I am *not* going to reveal the address of these two scientifically-minded females to anyone! However, I'm grateful to them for demonstrating that British women do have a sense of humour about sex (even in Leicester).

Q I do not reach multiple orgasms. Perhaps you could discuss the subject of oral sex, which more and more men seem to expect. **Common sense tells me that all forms of it must be unhygienic.**

A Common sense doesn't say anything of the kind, ma'am. It is certainly foolish to go in for oral sex when you have a mouth infection – or indeed, a sex infection.

It is particularly important not to do it when you have a 'cold sore' on the lip, as the virus which causes this is very nearly identical with the one which causes genital herpes.

But vast numbers of women do find oral love-play helpful in giving them orgasms (whether single or multiple), and enriching their sex lives generally. I can't see anything wrong with that.

Q I noticed your recent comment (in the **SHE** sex survey) about some women reaching orgasm when having their nipples touched.

Surely this is impossible?

I have never attempted to stimulate my wife in this way, because I have always assumed that her breasts (being small) are unresponsive.

A Small breasts are just as sexually responsive as big ones, sir

ORGASM

– so why not give it a go? I'm sure your wife would be pleasantly surprised – after all these years of not having her boobs touched!

I must stress that only a *tiny minority* of women can reach a climax in this way.

But an American survey of 'easily orgasmic women' revealed that 20% of these highly climactic females could 'come' just though having their nipples stroked or licked.

Q How on earth can you fake an orgasm! Surely a man must feel whether the vagina contracts or not at the moment of climax?

A First, I'm afraid that quite a few women do 'fake orgasm'. Regrettably, some doctors still advise them do to it – which I think is crazy.

In fact, it's quite easy to fake a climax. You see you're mistaken in thinking that at the moment of orgasm, the vagina contracts and so gives a signal to the man that climax has occurred. (Several other readers who're written to me have the same erroneous idea.)

Actually, it's extremely difficulty for a man to know with certainty whether a woman has reached a climax. Most men rely on a sort of hopeful guesswork – based on whether their partner's shrieks/groans/moans/whatever appear to be on a *crescendo* or not.

Alas, much of the sexual misunderstanding between male and female is due to the simple fact that many men simply haven't a clue as to whether their partners have 'done it'! Sometimes it's very difficult for gentlemen to follow the ancient rule 'Ladies come first...'

Q Re orgasm: I thought some of your readers might take comfort from my story. I am now 25, and for seven years I experienced frustration and depression because I could not 'come'.

At first I faked –though that's difficult when you don't known what you're supposed to be faking – but eventually I resigned myself to the non-event.

However, early last year, the big event *did* happen and afterwards all I could do was cry!

I now enjoy orgasm regularly, and my sex life with my husband is getting better and better. So my message to women is: don't give up.

A That's my message too. Thank you for a delightfully cheery letter. I think it's very important for

ORGASM

people to realise that the chances of reaching orgasm increase steadily as a woman gets older. Indeed, the graph is still climbing upwards at age 45, so no woman should ever lose hope.

Q My husband and I don't reach a simultaneous climax. Is this abnormal?

A Stone the crows, ma'am! The Delvin Report showed conclusively that only a minority of **SHE** readers usually 'come' at the same moment as their partners. Contrary to what so many 'bodice-ripper' novels would have us believe, simultaneous orgasm is really not all that common. So you're normal.

Q My fiancée does not reach orgasm during actual intercourse because she says my penis is too small. This is very distressing for me.

A I'm sure it is – and it's very unfortunate that she used this phraseology.

In fact, it's very unlikely that your penile size is anything to do with it. As I keep endlessly saying, most women do NOT regularly reach a climax during intercourse itself. So I think the two of you should go to a Family Planning Clinic and ask for: (a) some advice about love play; (b) a 'second opinion' on your phallic dimensions.

Q My problem is that I don't know if I've ever had an orgasm.

A If you don't know – then you haven't. Sorry to be so blunt! But from the rest of your letter, you're obviously very young and not very experienced sexually.

As I've often indicated, it's quite common not to have an orgasm until you've been established for some time in a relationship with a skilled and loving partner. Your day will come. (And so will you.)

Q This is not really a problem, more of a request for information. Should you not believe what I say, then I do not blame you. Some years ago I found out by accident that I could give a woman an orgasm just by holding her hand and using my mind. Later, I progressed to doing it just by holding the tip of a woman's finger and concentrating. And I even found that just by looking

ORGASM

into a woman's eyes. I could make her have an orgasm. Is this a common occurrence, or not?

A No, it's not common – even in Bournemouth, where you're writing from!

Frankly, sir, I'm a little doubtful whether you're serious. But if you really do think you can make women have climaxes just by gazing into their eyes, then I think you should ask yourself whether they're convulsing with orgasms – or with laughter.

Q I can't reach a climax, simply because my stupid husband refuses to accept that he has to stroke my clitoris in order to make me come!

He says that rubbing a woman's clitoris is 'unmanly' and maintains that women ought to be able to climax through intercourse, without any use of the hands. What can I do?

A Alas ma'am, many men have this delusion – which is why we've included a question on this very subject in our national survey of blokes.

But chaps who are well-read on the subject of the clitoris (I s'pose you could call them the *cliterati*, really) are aware that most women do need skilled manual stimulation of this organ if they are to reach orgasm easily.

Try showing this answer to your thick-witted, obstinate husband. If he *still* won't oblige, then I'm afraid you may have to resort to masturbation or a vibrator.

Q You were wrong when you said that the best indicator that a woman has reached orgasm is her loud cry.

You clearly don't know what you're talking about!

My vagina throbs such a lot that I'm sure any man could feel it and know that I've reached a climax.

A Well, I'm sorry to say that you're mistaken.

It's surprisingly difficult for a man to tell whether his lady has 'come' – unless she cries out.

That's why so many women are successful in faking orgasm – and also why so many blokes keep saying to their lovers: 'Er . . . have you come yet, dear?'

You're quite right in saying that at orgasm, the vagina contracts (about 8 or 10 times – at roughly 0.8 second intervals).

But contrary to what you might think, these 'throbs' aren't easy for a chap to feel – especially as a

ORGASM

very sexually-knowledgeable woman may have been deliberately contracting her pelvic muscles powerfully during intercourse.

Laboratory experiments in America (where else?) do show that the changes which take place in a woman's body at the moment of orgasm are either a) not easy to detect; or b) very readily faked.

The main 'orgasm indicators' which have been discovered in these experiments are:

Breasts: soon after orgasm, the previously 'collapsed' nipples start standing out more.
Skin: in many fair-skinned women, a 'sex flush' appear shortly before orgasm – and disappears at the time of climax.
Fingers and toes: these often curl up at the moment of orgasm.
Bottom: the muscles of your rear end contract involuntarily two to five times – if the orgasm is very intense.
Womb: this contracts powerfully during orgasm, but it's too high to be detected by the man.

These orgasmic changes were first described by the US sexologists, Virginia Johnson and William Masters – who together observed about 5,000 climaxes during research in the lab. (After which they did the decent thing and got married!)

Q When I 'come' with my boyfriend, I wet myself. He is very understanding, saying it's natural and he doesn't mind. But I do!

A I don't believe there's anything you can do about it – so I think it'd be better for you to try and adopt his sensible attitude.

Very large numbers of women do produce a fluid at the moment of orgasm. There's a lot of controversy about the nature of this fluid – which may be urine, or a secretion produced by the famous female 'G-spot'.

What is not controversial is that it is natural for these women to 'ejaculate' at orgasm.

Also, do bear in mind that some men find this phenomenon a very considerable 'turn on' – and a useful indicator that the lady really has come (see below).

Q Men never seem to know whether I have reached orgasm or not. What is the best 'indicator' to tell them to look out for?

A The cry ! There are various other physiological signs of

ORGASM

reaching a climax, but you'd need to be a very sharp-eyed sexologist to notice them.

So if you want to tell your man that you've got there, shriek loudly! (It'd also be a help if you seized the first available moment to say 'I've come...')

Q I was astounded to discover that most women don't reach a climax during intercourse.

I always do, and my husband and I *often* climax simultaneously. We have been married for 16 years, and I can count on one hand the number of times I haven't climaxed.

I thought that what we experienced was common to most couples. So it was only after reading your column that I realised how incredibly lucky we are.

A Too right. Until very recently, everybody from psychiatrists to readers of romantic fiction seemed to assume that most women automatically reached orgasm during intercourse itself – usually at the same time as their blokes did.

But the famous American sex researcher Ms Shere Hite (author of *The Hite Report*) rocked everybody by discovering that only about 30% of US women regularly reached orgasm during actual intercourse.

Since then, several large British surveys run by newspapers and magazines have shown that the figure for this country is about 30% to 40%.

However, I'd like to make clear that this *doesn't* mean that the rest of the female population aren't having an orgasm at all. It's just that they're mainly reaching it through love play.

Q I'm a mother of five children, and I'm extremely embarrassed by the fact that when I climax with my husband, I pass wind! Any ideas?

A Quite a common complaint – mainly due to the way the pelvic muscles tend to become slack after childbirth.

You may not be able to defeat your orgasm-flatulent problem completely. But 'pelvic' floor exercises might well help you to achieve better control over your wayward bottom?

Fortunately, the pelvic exercises which **SHE** popularised in conjuction with the self-help group SHAPE are now being taught in gyms and fitness studios.

I suggest you go along to the

ORGASM

nearest one and get yourself a pelvic toning-up course.

Q Can it really be true that some women are able to reach orgasm just through having their nipples rubbed! My husband says he once knew a girl who could do this, but I don't believe him.

A Well, ma'am, I do believe him – because it can happen.

But the ability to reach a climax through breast stimulation alone is unusual. So there's no need for you to feel inadequate because you can't peform the same difficult feat.

Q Whenever my partner and I make love, I find that the pressure tickles my bladder. So, if love-making carries on too long, I have to stop to go to the loo. I'd be grateful for any suggestions.

A Common problem, ma'am, I'm afraid. I think that all you can do is try to switch to other positions, in which the male organ doesn't press on the bladder or the urinary pipe.

One such posture is the 'lateral' in which your guy lies on his left side next to you, while you lie on your back with thighs raised – often known as 'having a bit on the side'.

Another useful trick would be to make sure that you remember to spend a penny before you start to make love, so that your bladder is completely empty.

Q Until just lately, I had a girl-friend in our town who claimed to reach 25 orgasms in a night – and she certainly *seemed* to when I was in bed with her. This was all a bit much for me, and we recently split up. But I wonder – was she faking?

A I doubt it. Though most women are happy with just one climax, there are quite a few who can knock off 20 or 25 in a session. You, sir, did very well to help her achieve such figures – and you've nothing to be ashamed of if she got a bit much for you to handle. (Note to male readers: no, gentlemen, I am not revealing any clues as to where this talented female resides.)

PASSING WIND

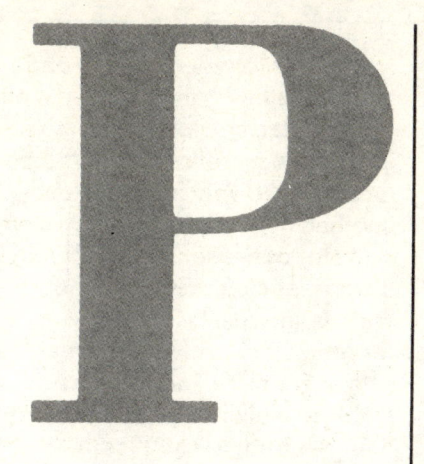

Q I have always regarded myself as a very feminine and fastidious woman, so I am distressed by something I can't seem to control. It is very embarrassing, and it's this – I can't help passing wind in bed, specially when making love. What can I do?

A Well, I'm not going to joke about this, because it can be a very upsetting problem. I've had a number of letters from women who are troubled by 'the wind', especially during pregnancy.

The only anti-gas measures I know of are the following:

cut right down on any fibre-containing food, including peas, beans and almost anything advocated by the F-Plan (!) Diet

try nibbling charcoal biscuits – these are obtainable without prescription from many chemists

if possible, sit on the loo for a good ten minutes before you go to bed – particularly if love-making is contemplated

But honestly, I think the most important thing is to talk this over with your man. If you can both laugh about it – rather than taking it seriously – then it will cease to matter.

PELVIC FLOOR

Pelvic Floor

What put me in mind of this structure was a conversation I had with an intelligent and well-informed woman who thought that pelvic floor exercises were so-called because you had to do them on the floor.

The pelvic floor is a sort of cleverly-interwoven basket of muscle which forms a network that supports all the organs in your pelvis – including your womb, your ovaries and your bladder.

You can get a rough idea of the size and shape of the muscles of the pelvic floor by simply holding your two hands palms upwards in front of you. Then slide the two hands together, so that the fingers interlock. The resulting shallow 'basin' is quite like the pelvic floor. Imagine that it's supporting your pelvic organs – and imagine too that (as in the anatomical drawing) there are two apertures in the 'basin', through which pass the vagina and the rectum.

Now it's important that all women should know about this pelvic floor musculature. Why? Because in so many, many females, childbirth leads to serious *weakening* of these muscles – with unfortunate consequences for your love-life and your health.

Repeated childbirth and *prolonged* or *difficult* labours are particularly likely to do this to a mother.

As far as her sex life is concerned, she's likely to find that her vagina seems to have become slack and loose. Either she or her bloke (or both) are liable to feel dissatisfied because things aren't as 'snug' as they once were.

The second consequence of pelvic floor slackness may be on the woman's health. After some years, severe weakness of these muscles can lead to prolapse (descent of the womb); much more frequently it simply causes problems with urination the woman finds that she has embarrassing incontinence, especially when she coughs or laughs.

Happily, gross weakness of the pelvic floor muscles can usually be put right with one of a variety of surgical 'repair operations'. But obviously, it's much better to avoid surgery altogether, and this can be done by means of pelvic floor exercises.

Every woman should do these exercises daily for several months after the birth of a child, in order to prevent prolapse and the other troubles I've men-

PELVIC FLOOR

tioned. Even when you've *already* got a good deal of pelvic floor weakness, its amazing how six months of Kegel exercises alone can often put things right. Ideally, every newly-delivered mother ought to be taught the exercises I'm going to describe. And any woman who feels that her vagina is a little too loose can do them too; they're quite good fun and they may prevent you from needing a vaginal 'repair' operation later on in life.

The exercises are called 'Kegel exercises', after the bloke who invented them.

The two exercises can and should be done during intercourse: this is enjoyable, for both of you. Why? Because once you've got these 'love muscles' developed a bit, you'll discover that doing the exercises creates an agreeable sort of 'milking' sensation in his male organ. (You don't get this kind of advice in other books, you know!)

But its no good just doing the two exercises during lovemaking. As with any other 'muscle building' exercises, you need to do them for about 20 minutes, twice a day – over at least six months. But here's the good news: you can do the exercises while you're at work, while you're pushing a pram, while you're sitting in the bath, while you're talking to the vicar, or whatever – no-one will know.

Exercise one: make a real effort to contract the *front* part of your pelvic muscles, by 'tightening up' as if you were trying to stop yourself passing water. Hold the contraction for ten seconds, then release for ten seconds, for ten minutes.

Exercise two: make a similar effort to contract the *back* part of your pelvic floor muscles by 'tightening up' as if to hold back a bowel movement. Again, maintain the contraction for ten seconds, then relax for ten. Repeat for ten minutes.

There are now at least four devices which are supposed to help people do Kegel exercises. The Gynatone is an acrylic vaginal cylinder to which you can attach successively greater weights as your vaginal muscles become stronger (seriously!). The Femtone is a simple isometric vaginal exerciser. Its makers also produce two much more complicated biofeedback-type devices; one of them converts your vaginal muscle contractions into electrical impulses and records them on a chart – and the other (incredibly enough) plays them back to you on a loudspeaker.

The Penis

The penis the organ which is the subject of an amazing amount of emotion and embarrassment and even outrage. Strange really, because it's a somewhat unimpressive little structure, comparing rather unfavourably in dimemsions with a decent-sized *andouillette*.

However, one has to face the fact that many men and women do have hang-ups about the penis. In the case of men, vast numbers of them have an extraordinary obsession about penile *size*.

In the case of women, a surprising number of females feel frightened or disgusted by the idea of a close encounter with a male organ. Some wives are so emotional about this matter that they cannot touch their husband's penises.

So it seems to me that life would be a great deal easier if everybody understood a few of the basic facts about this organ and how it works. Here goes!

The penis is the male equivalent of a woman's clitoris. So it's equipped with a great many pleasure receptors which, when stimulated, produce very agreeable sensations in the brain.

Now the average penis in its non-erect state is quite a bit smaller than most people imagine. Your average bloke measures between just over three inches (8.5 cm) and just over four (10.5 cm) when he's in this state – but it varies a lot, depending on the weather.

And the US sex researchers Masters and Johnson have discovered a curious fact of which few men are aware. Though penises vary quite a bit in size in the non-erect state, they're nearly all about the same size when they're erect – six and a half inches. So though many males feel inadequate about the size of their phalluses, this is all quite unnecessary – especially as most women aren't remotely interested in the size of a man's organ anyway.

The penis is a very simple structure in comparison with the female genital organ. Really it just consists of three cylinders of tissue, which are capable of filling with blood (thus causing an erection) when a man thinks about sex.

On the end of these three cylinders is the cone-shaped glans, which is the most sexually sensitive part. Hence the phrase: 'The Devil makes work for idle glans . . . ' Really, the only other thing to say about the penis is

PENIS SIZE

that contrary to what so many women (and men) imagine, it is actually a pretty *clean* structure. Provided a man washes regularly under his foreskin (if present) there should be nothing 'dirty' about his penis at all.

Amputation of the Penis

First, some good news. A treatment is now available for one of the most tragic accidents which can befall a boy or a man.

Because it's a somewhat vulnerable part of the body, the male organ can all too easily be chopped off in an accident. Also a few boys are born without the organ, and some men lose it through cancer or burns.

But at the East Virginia Medical School in America, plastic surgeons have developed a technique for fashioning a penis out of skin flaps taken from other parts of the body.

The method enables the patient to feel at least some sensation from his new penis. In one case, the establishment of sensation in the new organ has been so good that the young man in question has been able to achieve intercourse and even orgasm.

At the time of writing, I'm not aware that the operation has been attempted in Britain.

Q Is it really true that sex feels different if you do it with someone of another race?

A Not as far as I am aware. There are many myths about this – some of which, alas, are part of the obscene folklore of racial prejudice.

From a purely medical point of view, I'd say that I've noticed no structural differences between the sex organs of all the various races, so there's no particular reason why it should feel different.

Q We are three hairdressers in Exmouth, and we (and our customers) are a bit bewildered by the connection between a man's sexual performance the size of his penis.

So what we want to know is this: what is normal size? Please enlighten us, or we'll be forced to get out our rulers.

A I don't think that's a good idea! But many readers have written in saying they don't know what average size is. So here are the full, unexpurgated figures.

The average chap usually measures about three and a half

PENIS SIZE • PERVERSION

inches (that's 9 cm) in the resting condition — but much less in January because it's so chilly (even down in Exmouth).

When erect, the average bloke's measurement is six and half inches (16½ cm).

In fact, sexologists have been able to discover that 'resting' measurements are pretty irrelevant — because most penises tend to be very roughly the same size when they're erect, give or take an inch or two.

Now I would like to make one very serious point.

Most women are not aware of the fact that the average chap goes through life feeling a bit sexually inadequate because he's convinced his organ is on the small side. Even gentlemen equipped with eight inches (20.5 cm) or more can have this delusion!

Indeed, I actually get letters from guys terrified to take off their clothes in front of a woman — in case she laughs. There are chaps whose sex lives have been blighted permanently because somebody once thoughtlessly said to them: 'Your willy's not very big, is it?'

So dear readers, do try and avoid making that kind of morale-crumbling remark! We are, after all, an insecure and vulnerable sex...

Q I am a girl of 18, and I just keep feeling very dirty and guilty because of the fact that when I was about 11 or 12, I let my brother play around with me. Does this make me perverted?

A Not at all. There's a vast amount of this sort of childish experimentation around, so you're not abnormal in any way.

The best thing would be to forget all about it. But if it keeps preying on your mind, go and have a chat with your local *Brook Advisory Centre for Young People*.

Perversion

Different people mean entirely different things by this word. It's been shown that where a person hasn't had very much education, he's more likely to regard perfectly normal sexual activity as being 'wrong'. Even today, there are quite a few people around who think that any lovemaking between husband and wife other than intercourse in the 'standard' position is 'perverted'.

However, most people are rather better-informed than this, and the necessity for various types of love-play between husband and wife is generally recognized. Doctors in the field of sexual medicine do not regard any mutually-satisfying activity which is not harmful as being 'perverted'.

Psychological Illnesses

There are, however, true perversions, some of which are physically dangerous – sadism, masochism, and so on. A characteristic feature of all these is that the patient only wants satisfaction through his or her deviation and not through intercourse. Quite obviously, these are psychological illnesses which should be treated by a psychiatrist, if the patient will agree. (If he *won't* agree and you think he's dangerous, then ditch him –fast!)

Pheromone Production

'Wot on earth are pheromones?' I hear you cry.

Well, they're sex scents, actually. And they're pronounced '*fear*—oh-mones'.

They're delicate aromas which we all produce – so delicate in fact, that other people are scarcely (if at all) conscious of receiving them.

Yet their influence on other folk's sexual behaviour is said to be profound. For instance, the woman who produces a lot of female pheromones is believed to exert an unusually strong attraction on men.

And vice versa: the bloke who produces a lot of male pheromones may have what seems to be an inexplicable charm for women.

It's an interesting theory. And it may explain why in any gathering, there are certain people who are not especially beautiful or handsome in a physical way – yet who seem to be irresistible to the opposite sex.

Pheromones certainly play a very important sexual role in the rest of the animal kingdom. A lot of creatures are drawn to their potential mates by these scents.

Indeed, the most extreme example of pheromone attraction occurs in the pre-mating behaviour of the Emperor moth (*Eudia pavonia*). According to the estimable annual reference

PHEROMONE PRODUCTION • POSITIONS

work published by Messrs Guinness, the female puts out a pheromone which can be detected by the amorous male at the almost unbelievable distance of 6.8 miles! Human pheromones do not travel such vast distances, but are said to be able to exert their attraction across the proverbial crowded room.

It's not entirely clear which parts of the body produce them, but most are said to be generated by tiny glands in the genital, mouth and armpit areas.

In recent years, shrewd manufactures have 'bottled' male and female pheromones – extracted from animals – in aerosol sprays. These are now quite widely advertised in classified columns and amazing claims are made for their alleged attractant powers. The makers claim that if you spray male pheromones on certain chairs in a room, all the woman who come in will choose those chairs.

Unfortunately, the only demonstration I've ever seen of this alleged effect ended in a complete shambles – mainly because the demonstrator was so plastered that he couldn't remember which chairs he'd sprayed with what.

However, whether the commercially produced pheromone aerosols really do work or not, there seems to be reasonable evidence that the woman who produces a lot of female pheromone is unusually attractive to men.

Q My sex life with my fiancé is fantastic, but I only climax when I'm making love astride him. This worries me.

A You're very lucky to be able to reach a climax during intercourse at all. Be glad of this! When you're married a few years, you'll probably find that climaxes will result from other positions too.

Q I'm about to have a hip replacement. My husband and I used to like to complete our lovemaking with me sitting on him, but at present I can't because of pain. Will it be possible again once I've had the op?

A Almost certainly, ma'am, if the op goes well (as it usually does). P'raps you'd like to write

POSITIONS

and tell me if you've been able to get back to your old position again?

You might like to know that the French call your favourite posture 'La Diligence de Narbonne' ('The Narbonne Stagecoach') – because of the powerful bumping sensation it produces.

Q I get tremendous pleasure from being made love to 'doggie-fashion' by my husband. Am I abnormal? Is it perhaps that it's because I was born in the Year of the Dog?

A Is it perhaps that you're sending me up, ma'am? Anyway, there's nothing wrong with making love in this way if you want to.

Admittedly, it's not the most romantic of positions (and in my personal view, it's not exactly the most dignified either). But a lot of people find it satisfying. And some women find it more comfortable than the more 'usual' positions.

Q For various reasons, I cannot tolerate my husband making love to me while lying on top of me, face-to-face. My doctor has suggested that a rear entry position would solve the problem, but somehow I feel that this is too 'animal' for me. Have you any suggestions?

A Indeed yes. Many couples find that the face-to-face missionary position doesn't suit – for instance, because the woman is advanced in pregnancy, or because the husband is much heavier than her, or (quite frequently) because the woman feels threatened or unable to control things in this traditional face-to-face posture.

Similarly, many women are unhappy about 'rear entry' positions – which are a little too reminiscent of your friendly neighbourhood spaniel and his hobby for some people's tastes.

The solution lies in the fact that there are literally countless other positions (which surprisingly few couples know about, but which are detailed in text-books on the subject). For example, an excellent and comfortable compromise can be found in the celebrated 'left lateral position' – in which the woman lies on her back with her knees bent, while her man lies on his side alongside her, entering from behind her thighs. This is sometimes jokily known as 'having a bit on the side'.

'Tomorrow,' as Milton so sagaciously remarked in *Lycidas*, 'to fresh woods and postures new'.

POSITIONS

Positions

How Many Positions Are There?

One of the nice things about making love is the fact that there are lots and lots of different ways of doing it. You can make love in a wide variety of ways, and so give each other all sorts of differing pleasant sensations.

How many different ways are there? People are forever arguing about this; one person will say with absolute assurance that there are 71 – while another will announce that the ancient Persians discovered no less than 423.

What's the truth? The fact is that there's no *exact* number of positions. It would be possible to make up a list of hundreds and hundreds provided that you were willing to accept that there were only very minor differences between some of them.

It's also important to remember that some of the wilder antics described in certain books are either dangerous or quite impossible for anyone but a pair of Olympic gymnasts. To take an extreme instance, the oft-quoted example of making love 'swinging from a chandelier' is clearly utter nonsense. (One wonders how many aristocratic families have ruined their best light fixtures this way . . .)

On a more practical level, some of the 'man leaning back' positions mentioned in certain ancient texts are very likely to strain a man's spine – and possibly fracture his penis too! I jest not. Leaning back too far while making love can have disastrous consequences. But rest assured that all the positions mentioned in this chapter are quite safe.

Why Bother with All These Different Positions Anyway?

That's a good question. And the fact is that if you're happy making love in just one single position, and both of you are perfectly satisfied, then that's fine! Carry on doing it the same way.

But the fact is that most people do like a reasonable amount of variety in their love-making. They find that trying out various positions prevents dullness creeping in. (And dullness is something that can cause a lot of problems in marriage.)

They also find that trying out something different gives them all sorts of pleasant new

POSITIONS

sensations. Sometimes these sensations can help a woman to respond far better than she did before. Sometimes too, they will even help her reach a climax – when previously she had difficulty in doing so.

Furthermore, some women find that sex in an 'ordinary' position is uncomfortable or even painful. (This is particularly common when the male partner is much heavier than the wife.) In these circumstances, a change to an alternative position may well solve the problem.

Incidentally, women who have a 'retroverted' womb – that is, one that points backwards – sometimes find that they have to try out all sorts of love-making positions before they discover one that's really comfortable.

But the main reason why people do like to try out different positions is that it just happens to be fun...

Love-making Positions and Fertility

Does the position in which you make love affect your chances of getting pregnant? There are two points to bear in mind here.

Firstly, a lot of people still have the idea that if you make love in a standing position, then pregnancy is impossible. This is nonsense – you can start a baby in any position.

But the second point is very important for couples who have difficulty in conceiving. If your fertility is as bit below par and you're trying for a baby, you should take care to choose love-making positions which give the man's sperm the best possible chance of entering the womb.

For instance, a woman whose womb is retroverted stands the best chance of getting pregnant if she makes love in one of the 'face down' positions described later in this chapter.

This is because a 'face down' position will make the neck of her womb dip into the pool of sperm which forms at the top of her vagina after her partner has reached his climax.

Many infertility clinics advise women with retroverted wombs to have intercourse on all fours, with the man behind them – and to stay in this admittedly somewhat undignified posture for about 10 minutes afterwards.

In contrast, women whose wombs point in the normal direction are usually advised by infertility clinics to have sexual intercourse in one of the 'face up' positions – preferably with a couple of pillows under her

POSITIONS

bottom, so as to encourage the sperm to stay at the top of the vagina, in contact with the neck of the womb.

Love-making Positions, Arthritis and Disability

From my problem page postbag, I have learned over the years that knowledge of a variety of love-making positions can be a surprising help to people with arthritis, as well as to people with certain other disabilities.

For instance, it's very common for a woman who has arthritis of the hips, but who is otherwise still fit and sexy, to find that the pain and stiffness in her hips make it impossible for her to lie back and make love in the traditional or 'missionary' positon.

A lot of women who have this problem have written to me asking if there's any other position which wouldn't give them pain. Very frequently, a simple change to, say, the 'Spoons' position is enough to solve the problem.

Similarly, men and women who are disabled by back problems, or even by paralysis of a limb, often find that they can still make love with their partners by choosing a position in which their disability is no longer a handicap.

To take one light-hearted example, I can remember a woman who had broken both her legs, and who therefore had to spend several months with her two lower limbs immobile in plaster. She was, however, very keen on making love with her husband – and she managed to continue to do it regularly by going in for an energetic version of the 'cross-buttock' position position described later in this section.

Love-making Positions and Pregnancy

The one time when vast numbers of women really do need to try out other positions is during pregnancy.

From about the middle of pregnancy onwards, it becomes increasingly difficult for a woman to bear the weight of a man on her tummy. These days, many couples make love far into the eighth or even ninth month of pregnancy. And at *that* stage, sex in the missionary position is getting perilously near to impossible.

Mothers-to-be are therefore well advised to try out some of the positions to which I have indicated as being good in pregnancy in this section – particularly those in which the

POSITIONS

man enters from the side or from behind.

The Positions Most Likely to Give Happiness

In a moment we'll embark on the list of positions which I've chosen for this book. They are, in my view, the positions which are most likely to give a loving couple a good deal of pleasure and happiness.

But if you're repelled or appalled by a particular posture (for instance, some people have a deep aversion to all 'rear entry' positions because of their canine associations), then you shouldn't bother with it: move on to something else instead.

What you'll *not* find in this section are daft, dangerous or impossible positions – though I must admit that it's a bit of a temptation to include one or two of the more bizarre ones I have encountered in my researches.

Face to Face, with Man Above

The first and most common position of love-making is of course the so-called 'missionary' position – the one in which the woman lies flat on her back with her knees raised, while the man lies between her thighs.

This is a pleasant and comfortable position which suits most people very well. Most important is the obvious fact that the couple can kiss each other on the lips while making love. They can also talk to each other – something which isn't terribly easy with the more exotic postures!

Sex books always allege that the history of the position's name is that the white missionaries of Victorian days recommended it to their native converts. I've no idea whether this is true – but if so, I think it says a great deal for the good sense of the missionaries! For this is a very nice, warm, snuggly position, with what sexologists like to call 'a good degree of penetration'.

There are, however, a couple of drawbacks to the missionary position. One is that it's a little difficult for the man to reach the woman's clitoris with his fingertips. (So if it's important to you to have your clitoris stimulated during love-making, you might like to try some of the 'rear entry' positions described later in this section.

The other drawback is that if the man is much heavier than the woman, the missionary posture can be quite uncomfortable, or

POSITIONS

even painful, for her. The same may be true if she's pregnant. In these circumstances, a sideways or rear entry position my be both more comfortable and more fun.

Finally, I ought to mention that a surprising number of men do have a bit of trouble with the missionary position because they lose their erections just as they try to get 'on top'.

A woman should bear in mind that a man who's a little uncertain about his erection may perform better if he's flat on his back.

Variations on the Missionary Position

A very good idea is to put a couple of pillows under your bottom, so as to tilt it upwards. This decidedly alters the sensations which you and your partner will experience in the missionary position, mainly because you'll find that penetration is deeper. Putting a hot-water bottle under the woman's buttocks has a similar effect.

The next position is *Toulouse*. It's very similar to the missionary position – except that the man's legs are *outside* the woman's. This may seem a rather trivial point, but in fact, the sensations produced by this position are rather different. And – very important – the position is quite useful for the many women who find that child-bearing has made their vaginas lax. This is because the fact that the woman's thighs are *inside* the man's enables her to use her thigh muscles to hold him more snugly – which is nicer for both of them, as a rule.

A thid position in this group is *Béziers*. It's really very like the missionary position – except that the woman spreads her legs out as widely as possible. A lot of ladies find a great deal of sensuous pleasure from this cat-like, 'stretching' position.

Women who own four-poster beds may actually curl their feet around the bedposts. And couples who have a liking for mild forms of bondage may actually go in for tying the woman's ankles to the bedposts. (*Warning*: bondage is most certainly *not* everybody's cup of tea.)

The next 'face to face with male above' position is *Bagnères*. This is a natural development of the missionary position – except that the lady missionary brings her legs up and wraps them round the man's waist.

The lady has to be fairly fit and supple to be able to do this, but the resulting position is good fun

POSITIONS

for both partners. The altered tilt of the woman's pelvis will usually produce interesting new sensations for both of them.

And so on to *Avignon* where once again, the woman has her legs wrapped round her man's waist – but here he has to *kneel* on the bed (or whatever). If the man is a trifle too enthusiastic there's a slight tendency for his repeated thrusts to keep banging the lady's skull against the headboard of the bed; however, this can be guarded against by skilful placing of the pillows.

The *Narbonne* position is similar but, the man now kneels on the floor behind her, while she (also kneeling) rests her top on the edge of the bed or whatever.

Once again, the over-enthusiastic lover must take care not to be too violent – or he may propel both bed and partner straight across the room and into the nearest wall.

The *Bordeaux* position is an interesting one, but only suitable for the woman with a really supple spine. Lying on her back on the bed, the lady draws her legs up really far, so that she's able to put them over the man's shoulders.

This somewhat exotic position will almost certainly give her all sorts of unusual and even bizarre sensations. The man will probably quite enjoy it too. He should take things very gently, because penetration is very deep indeed in this position.

This position is probably best avoided in late pregnancy, because of the depth of penetration achieved. And I certainly wouldn't recommend it for the sexually inexperienced woman, who might quite reasonably take fright at being asked to assume such an acrobatic pose.

Last in this 'Face to face, male superior' group is the *Montois*, in which the man lies with his body across the woman's, and at 90° to it. In this position, the woman may achieve various interesting sensations, because the man's penis is pressing against the *side* of her vagina. In a variation on this position, the man only turns his body through 45 instead of 90 degrees. This is somewhat improbably known as the 'half cross-buttock'.

Face to Face, with Woman Above

Now we come to the first group of 'female superior' positions. There are still a few men who think that these positions are somehow demeaning to the dignity of the male sex – but I'm

POSITIONS

sure that their opinions may be safely discounted.

Let's begin with the simple *La Voulte* position. The woman lies on top of the man – in this case with her legs outside his.

This is really a most comfortable position, particularly if the woman is much lighter than her partner. Men appreciate it too – especially as there's a sort of suggestion that the female is seducing the male by making love to him in this way.

To get into this position, all you really need do is this. First, make sure your partner has an erection (sounds silly, but you'd be surprised at how often this elementary preliminary is neglected), then gently throw a leg across his thighs, and climb on top – if necessary, using your hand to guide him in.

In an obvious variation of this position, the woman has her legs *inside* the man's. This is *Carcassonne*. As with the equivalent 'male superior' position this position gives a snug fit – which may be helpful to the couple if the woman's pelvic muscles are a little loose because of childbearing.

Another useful 'female superior' position is *Brive*. It's also called the 'frog' – and I *think* I christened this myself in an earlier book of mine (though if somebody else thought of the name first, I apologize). I hasten to add that the expression 'frog position' has no Gallic overtones, and isn't meant to imply that this particular posture is favoured in the land of the can-can. It just means that you both spread your legs in a breast stroke-type way, so that your pubic regions are pushed together. This is another of those positions which isn't specially romantic, but does often give extremely good sexual sensations.

Another extremely useful female superior position is *Perpignan*. Its quite easy for a woman to get into this position by simply kneeling down *astride* her man, (who is lying flat on his back).

Now this position is very nice but why do I call it 'useful'? Simply because couples who have minor or even major sex difficulties are often advised to try it. The main reason for this is that the position puts no pressure on the woman: if (as is very common) she's a little frightened of intercourse, or tends to panic when the tip of a penis enters her body, then this position leaves her *in control*. She can withdraw a little whenever she wants to – and in effect take charge of the

POSITIONS

whole act of love if that's what she feels happiest with.

It's easy to develop other positions from this one: for instance, the woman can put one or indeed both legs out to the side (depending how supple she is), and so vary the sensations she feels.

Women who are good at yoga can cross their legs in front of them – across the man's chest. It's even possible to adopt the famed 'lotus position' – though it might be as well to support yourself with your hands while you do this, for fear of falling over and perhaps giving your man a badly sprained penis!

The *Lyon* position is really just one stage on from *Perpignan*. The woman stretches her legs out in front of her, so that she's really sitting on him (facing him) as he lies on his back. She can really move about in the most amazing way in this position, giving both herself and the man a lot of pleasure.

Clearly, the woman can move herself from this position into several closely related ones – for instance, by turning her legs first through 45 degrees and then through 90 degrees in either direction. She can also turn to face away from the man, and then (if she likes) complete a full circle by returning to face him again.

I call the *Grenoble* position 'the lean back'. You can quite easily get into it from the *Lyon* position. All you have to do is to lean backwards, until your head touches the bed. This should give you very pleasant and unusual sensations, as your partner's penis presses against the *front* of your vagina – and against the famous G-spot.

But do go a bit gently as you lean back, because you are putting your partner's penis under a fair amount of tension. This ought to be very agreeable for him – but a *sudden* lean back could produce pain, and (if you were really violent about it) the ultimate disaster of a ruptured penis. I suppose there are some blokes who *deserve* that sort of thing, but I'm sure you wouldn't want to go to bed with them.

Exotically-minded lovers can find all sorts of variants of the lean back position, by simply trying out the effect of straightening out various legs, and seeing what happens.

Olympique de Paris is a much less ambitious position – and one which is quite easy for most couples, provided the man is moderately supple. First, look back to page 104, and then take

POSITIONS

up the ordinary female superior *Carcassonne* position described earlier. The man then raises his legs so that his thighs are alongside the woman's bottom. He can then raise them even further so that they're up around her waist – and he can even cross them behind her back.

This is a pleasant, abandoned sort of position, in which the man can repeatedly pull himself up into the woman, creating sensations which both of them will find agreeable.

Biarritz is what might be called the 'Half Cross Bum' position. It's another female superior position – but she turns herself through about 45 degrees on top of the man, a manoeuvre which will give her quite different sensations inside the vagina. This position does give the man a very good opportunity to caress her bottom (and, indeed her breasts if that's what she likes).

The 'Full Cross' or *Vienne* is really just a development of the last one. The woman turns through 90 degrees on top of the man, so that she's lying at right-angles to him. This certainly makes conversation difficult (which is why I give this posture such an abysmally low romance rating), but the effect on the erotic nerve endings can be quite gratifyingly startling.

Face to Face, Sitting

A lot of people like to make love sitting in a chair – though I'd recommend that you choose a nice, comfortable one, which isn't likely to collapse. I'm slightly baffled by books which suggest that couples should make love on deck-chairs; if you try it, do be very careful!

Association Sportive a pleasant face to face sitting position. The bloke sits on a kitchen chair or stool, and the lady just sits astride him, facing him. Some couples like to try out these chair positions first with their clothes on – since they feel that this is rather more risqué. Obviously, the woman just removes her pants and tights – or wears open-crotch ones.

Face to Face Standing

Stade Français involves a couple making love in a standing position, face to face. If you have been making love horizontally in bed for years, and need something new to make sex more varied, then this could be the answer.

Standing sex has had a bit of a bad press – mainly because it tends to be used for illicit love-

POSITIONS

making by young couples who have no bedroom to go to. But in fact it can be very pleasant.

Since men are usually a bit taller than their female partners its easier if the man can stand so that he's a little *lower* than his partner. If you're both on the same level, it can be a bit of a strain on the legs – and you may well find out why this position is often referred to as the 'dreaded knee-trembler'!

Racing Club is another version of face to face love-making while standing up. The man lifts the woman up so that she can wrap her legs round him. This is a most entertaining position, which tends to appeal to couples with a sense of humour – but it's best not attempted if the man has any back trouble.

Rear Entry

Now we move on to the 'rear entry' positions. Some people don't like these, because they consider them undignified and rather too close to what goes on in the animal world. But some rear entry positions can be very comfortable – particularly the 'Spoons' one, which we'll come to in a moment. Also, some of them are very practical during pregnancy.

Furthermore, these positions can help a lot of women who need extra clitoral stimulation during intercourse. For in a rear-entry position, one great advantage is the fact that it is easy for the man to reach round with his hand and stimulate the woman's clitoris with his fingertips. Quite often, this can help her achieve orgasm during intercourse when otherwise she wouldn't have done so.

Most common rear entry positions are practised with the man above. But it's also perfectly possible to make love rear entry-style with the woman above.

A very similar position, but this time on a chair, is the *Bègles*.

Then there's the 'Spoons' or *Dax* – a comfortable, cosy position. The couple lie on their sides on the bed, with the man snuggled up behind the woman. This is a nice way for a couple to cuddle up together on a cold winter's night – and perhaps fall asleep afterwards, their bodies curving harmoniously together like two spoons in a drawer. (This one is good in pregnancy too.)

Very sensuous are several variations on this theme. The first of these is similar to the Spoons – but with the woman bending the top half of her body right forward until it's at 90 degrees to

POSITIONS

the man's body. In a second variation, the man leans backwards. And similar to this last one is a third variation, in which the woman thrusts her leg backwards between the man's thighs, as far as it'll go. Surprisingly enough, this produces strikingly different and pleasant sensations.

Finally, one rear entry position which is worth trying is the standing one. The woman can 'develop' this by bending forward, if she wants to. If she's quite lithe and lissom, she may want to experiment with the sensations caused by bending very far forward until her hands touch the floor. Provided your lover isn't the sort of idiot who tries to drive your head through the carpet, this can be very agreeable. Also worth trying is bending forward over a comfortable sofa or armchair.

Q I am eight months pregnant, but still very much enjoy making love with my husband. Only trouble is, it's getting a bit uncomfortable now, what with my 'bump'!
Are there any positions which would be more comfortable?

A There are many, ma'am. Probably the most popular for expectant mums is the one in which you simply lie face to face on top of your husband.
This is known in the obstetric world as the 'Mother Superior' position...

Q Re: the position you described as 'having a bit on the side' my husband and I have attempted it, and we think it is impossible.

A You really must try harder, ma'am! All you have to do is lie on your back with knees raised. Your husband then lies on his side with his thighs curled up under your bottom. I'd come round and demonstrate, but I do not make house calls.

Premature Ejaculation

These days, increasing numbers of women are unwilling to put up with premature ejaculation ('hair-trigger trouble'). And a good thing too, in my opinion!

In the olden days (like about 1960), there was no effective treatment for this all-too-common male condition. Furthermore, women were willing to accept the fact that lots of guys could only 'manage it' for a couple of minutes. But today, it seems to me that the average Britoness demands much, much more! Certainly the latest figures suggest that the late 1980s woman isn't prepared to put up with sexual intercourse lasting only two or three minutes – she frequently prefers 15 or 20 minutes or more. So, if her mate is ejaculating too prematurely for her, she takes him along to the doc for treatment.

Hang on – before we get to treatment, why does premature ejaculation happen at all? Well, it does seem to me that some chaps are by nature rather explosively triggered – especially when they're young. But orthodox teaching says that most prematurely ejaculating males were *conditioned* by their early sexual experiences.

In other words, they first made love in situations, like the back of car, were they felt that they had to reach a climax fast – and they've gone on doing so ever since.

But the great thing is, nowadays you can treat your man's hair-trigger trouble.

For by far the most efficient way of treating 'PE' is the one developed by US sex researchers Johnson and Masters, who found that if a woman uses an 'orgasm delay grip' on her man, she can re-train him over a period of months, so that eventually he can last for as long as they both wish.

The exact explanation of the delay grip must be taught over several weeks by a Johnson and Masters therapist. (Ask your doc to refer you to one.)

The grip – which has to be very precise – involves placing your thumb on one part of your man's penis, and your index and middle fingers on the prescribed location on the opposite side. You then give a deft squeeze and the not-unpleasant sensation which this produces will stop him from reaching a climax.

It's rather like stopping a sneeze by pressing your upper lip – but a good deal more fun.

PREMATURE EJACULATION

Q I am married to a dentist who suffers from premature ejaculation. I have tried to put up with this over the years.

Unfortunately, he recently had what he thought was the brilliant idea of using some local anaesthetic ointment on his penis in order to reduce his sensitivity and slow him down. After he'd used it about half a dozen times, I suddenly got an intense redness and soreness of my vaginal opening, which has driven me nearly crazy.

I have been unable to make love at all since then. This is extremely frustrating for me, because in actual fact, what my husband doesn't know is that I have to obtain all of my sexual satisfaction through having an affair with his partner.

A I'm sorry to hear about this dreadful mess. As regular readers of my work will know, most cases of inflammation of the vulva are due to infection.

In case this is so, you should immediately go to a clinic or a doctor who is equipped to make the tests for the common genital infections.

But I suspect that what has happened here is that you've developed a violent 'sensitivity reaction' to your husband's ointment. This is very common with local anaesthetics, and I actually had such a reaction myself once – though only (I hasten to add) through using it for sunburn.

If it is a sensitivity reaction, your doc will probably treat you with anti-histamine pills.

When you've recovered, why don't you and your husband go along to a clinic which specialises in the more sensible way of treating premature ejaculation?

Q I love my fiancé very much, but he 'comes' almost as soon as he gets inside me. This has hit his confidence very badly. We are supposed to get married next year, but I am afraid that if this goes on, he will call everything off.

A Your fiancé is suffering from a very common male complaint called 'premature ejaculation' – which is also known as 'hair trigger trouble.'

There's a simple method of treatment called 'Masters-Johnson therapy.' If you and your chap go together to a Family Planning Clinic, they'll be able to point you in the direction of a therapist who specialises in this kind of problem.

Promiscuity

The fact has to be faced that promiscuous sexual behaviour has now become very widespread in young people – in women as well as in men.

Distinguished British sociologist Michael Schofield studied a large group of 25-year-olds, some of whom were married.

He found that:

almost one third of them had had *no* sex partners in the previous year

almost one third had had only *one* partner in a year

a tiny proportion had had just *two* partners in a year

but a full third had had *three or more* partners (sometimes many more) in the course of a year.

So Schofield found that nowadays a very large proportion of women and men in their early-to-mid twenties do go through a decidedly promiscuous phase. It cannot be denied that the rise in VD in western society – and the emergence of new and alarming types of sexually transmitted disease – is related to the fact that people do have many more partners these days.

Regrettably, there are a lot of men in this age group who have a quite extraordinarily aggressive appetite for sexual conquest, and who will quite cheerfully have sex with 200 partners per year or more, if let loose. Anyone with even a passing acquaintance with bacteriology will realize that this sort of foolish, irresponsible behaviour unfortunately provides a sort of perpetual Christmas party for germs!

Happily, most men and women who go through a rather promiscuous phase between about 20 and 26 do eventually get over it and settle down to a monogamous – or at least relatively monogamous – relationship which they intend to be life-long.

PROMISCUITY • PROSTATE GLAND

Q I am 26 and thinking of settling down and getting married. But one thing worries me. It's this: I counted up on my fingers the other day and found that I have had no less than 11 lovers. Do you think this makes me terribly promiscuous?

A No – but it does rather sound as if you have 11 fingers. Seriously, people do vary a great deal in the amount of sexual experience they've had. Recently I tried to reassure a woman of about the same age as yourself that it was perfectly normal for her to be a virgin. Similarly, by today's standards it's not very unsual for a 26-year-old to have slept with 11 men over (presumably) quite a few years. You seem to have survived these experiences, and I hope you enjoyed them.

Prostate Gland

The prostate gland is about the size of a chestnut. In fact, if you imagine a conker with a hole through, you'll have a good idea of what a prostate is like.

It's located just below the bladder. The urethra (or urinary pipe) runs straight through it. It's claimed that this makes it the exact embryological equivalent of the Famous Female G-Spot.

What does it *do*? Well, its only known function is a sexual one. It adds a fair old contribution to the fluid which a man ejaculates when he has a climax. The prostatic secretion is thought to give impetus to the sperms in some way – and the added volume probably does give a boost to his sensual satisfaction.

Disorders

There are two main problems with the prostate gland: *enlargement*, and *cancer*.

In most men, the gland increases markedly in size after about the age of 50. For fairly obvious reasons of 'plumbing', this tends to interfere with the water-works. Indeed, if the enlargement is too great, it may become impossible to pass urine.

PROSTATE GLAND • PUBIC HAIR

Prostate trouble is so common that two recent British prime ministers have had theirs removed. As an alternative to removal, there is a newer and milder operation called a 'TUR' in which part of the gland is nibbled away by a slim instrument pushed up the urinary pipe.

Cancer of the prostate is, of course, far more serious. It is treated (often successfully) by removal of the gland, plus hormone therapy and possibly radiation.

Stimulation

From a sexual point of view, prostatic stimulation is possible and (I gather) widely practised in the more exotic parts of the world.

It is done by gentle massage with a well-lubricated finger and tends to produce a more intense climax with a more powerful ejaculation. However, as the massage has to be via the gent's bottom, there are obviously hygenic risks involved.

Q I have blonde hair, which is natural, I might add. But my pubic hair is dark. and my lover wants me to dye it blonde. Would there by any harm in this?

A Well I certainly wouldn't do it because your bloke wants you to do it – only take the plunge if *you* fancy the idea of having blonde pubes.

Tinting your 'maidenhair' involves very little more risk than tinting the hair on your head. However, you should certainly do a test first – and of course drop the whole idea if you develop the slightest soreness or irritation.

But an adverse reaction is most unlikely, and you know what they say: blondes have more fun.

RAPE

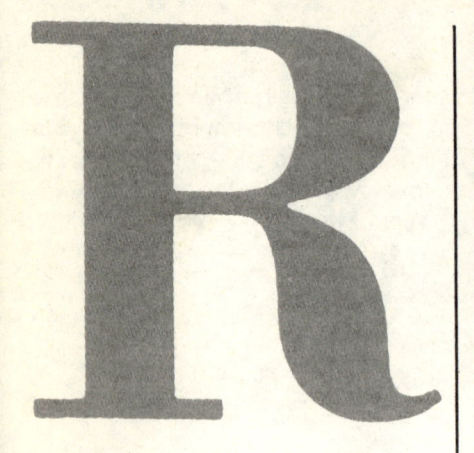

Rape

Rape is a hideous crime. In many cases, it's associated with terrifying violence. Some of the letters I've received in my postbag over the years from women who've been raped make it clear that being the victim of this sort of thing is a shattering experience which leaves the woman feeling dirty, degraded and (perhaps surprisingly) guilty.

And doctors who have treated rape victims are well aware that often they are psychologically scarred for life. Quite often, the ordeal that these women are subjected to is far more brutal and disgusting than you would guess from reading the reports in the newspapers.

Indeed, many cases are *never* reported in the papers – simply because a lot of women never report the attack to the police. This is partly due to a lack of confidence in the way the police will handle the matter.

Alas, it can't be denied that in Britain, Europe and America, police forces have a pretty abysmal record in dealing with women who have reported a rape. However, things *are* slowly improving – partly thanks to the widespread development of Rape Crisis Centres run by women.

RAPE

Avoiding Rape

Regrettably, no woman is entirely safe from rape – specially as it so often happens within the home. I've tried here to set out some guidelines on how to avoid rape; what to do if somebody attempts it; and what to do afterwards:

1 Don't walk along dark or lonely roads, or cross open ground when there's nobody about.
2 Be particularly wary at night – and especially in the hours after the pubs close (many rapes are alcohol-related).
3 At night, it's far better to take a cab than to walk – the expense may prevent you from having a dangerous experience (or even save your life).
4 Never accept lifts from men – especially late at night.
5 Never travel in single train compartments by yourself – pick an open compartment with other people in it, and sit near another woman.
6 Keep your doors and accessible windows locked, and put a chain on your front door.
7 If you *have* to go out at night, consider carrying a 'rape alarm' – a small canister that gives out a loud and alarming noise.
8 Attend self-defence classes for women.
9 If the law permits it in your country (it doesn't in Britain), consider carrying a weapon for defending yourself.

What to Do if You're Attacked

If a man, or group of men, starts being troublesome, you still have a good chance of avoiding rape. Follow the following rules.

1 At all costs, *don't look submissive* – women's anti-rape groups quite rightly teach that a woman who looks alert and ready to fight back may put the man off.
2 Yell for help – noise is a good deterrent and does actually frighten some men off.
3 Show active resistance: for instance, if a hand is put on you, grab the man's little finger (which is weak) and rip the hand away. Allowing a hand to remain on you will be interpreted as an invitation to go further.
4 If you think you have a reasonable chance of success, *fight back hard* – using any available methods (e.g. kicking him in the testicles, gouging him in the eye, ramming in a high heel or the tip of an umbrella).
5 As an alternative, it may be worth trying to *talk* your way out: some women have succeeded by striking up some sort of brief rap-

RAPE

port and getting the man to discuss his problems.
6 Don't forget devious ploys like pretending you have womb cancer or VD – these have saved some women in the past.
7 At the point when all seems lost, remember that a man with an erection can be disabled for five or 10 seconds by grasping his organ firmly and twisting it ferociously through about 90°.
8 If you do get free by violent methods, then for heaven's sake, *run*. (Kick off any high heels.) If you're caught again, you're going to get hurt.
9 If you're in fear of your life – e.g. if he has a gun or knife – then *give in*: at least you'll stay alive.
10 Finally, whatever happens, try to fix every detail about the rapist's appearance in your mind.

What to Do if You Have Been Raped

It's a terribly shocking experience, but do your best to follow these guidelines.

1 Get to a phone and ring a Rape Crisis Centre (Rape Control Centre) – these are organizations run by women in many large cities. You'll find the number in the telephone book. Even if the nearest number is far away, ring it (reverse the charges if necessary).
2 Do exactly as the people at the Rape Crisis Centre tell you.
3 Call the police: you may feel very much against the idea – but remember that if they catch the rapist, that should protect other women against his activities for quite a while.
4 *Don't* wash and *don't* change your clothes. If a conviction is to be secured, you'll have to have a forensic examination by a specially qualified doctor – and if you wash or change, the evidence will be gone.
5 Unless you're on the Pill or are otherwise protected against pregnancy, then within 24 hours of the rape make sure you find a doctor who will give you the morning-after Pill to prevent you from conceiving.
6 A week or so after being raped you should for your own protection, go to a doctor for preliminary VD tests (there's no point in going any earlier as the tests couldn't be positive).
7 If you become deeply disturbed as a result of what's happened, do keep in touch with the Rape Crisis Centre (01–837 1600) and don't hesitate to seek psychiatric help and counselling.

ROMANCE

Romance

Men in particular are all too likely these days to forget the importance of romance in a relationship. Regrettably, books, films and TV often picture sex as an emotionless business, in which people meet, leap into bed together, have intercourse, smoke a cigarette – and move on!

But real life can't be conducted at that level. We're not machines but deeply complex, emotional creatures who need to be cherished and loved. The man or woman who forgets that fact does so at his or her peril.

Romance, Emotion and Sexuality in Women

As Lord Byron remarked:
'Man's love is of man's life a thing apart,
'Tis woman's whole existence.'

As he implied, men would do well to remember that for a woman, love is usually a far more all-embracing, emotional and even spiritual business than it is for a man. Unfortunately, a man may regard sexual intercourse as far and away the most important aspect of a love relationship with a woman. But it's vital for him to realize that most women see life and love quite differently. A woman is *most* unlikely to view her relationship with a man in crude terms of a penis entering her vagina.

Instead, her view of the love relationship is likely to be bound up with such things as:

the warm glow she feels when he's around

the sense of being valued and wanted as a person by him

the feeling of rightness and completeness that comes from being one half of a loving couple.

If a man doesn't appreciate that his partner has this strongly romantic perception of the love relationship, then he may well be heading for trouble. Certainly, a vast number of marriages founder these days simply because the man fails to satisfy the woman's need for romance.

Romantic Tips for Men

What amazes me after so many years in the advice business is that again and again men go wrong because they fail to follow a few simple 'do's and don'ts'.

Do:
take the trouble to smarten yourself up before you meet her

ROMANCE

hold her hand

catch her eye and smile at her when you're in a crowd.

compliment her on her appearance

tell her she smells nice

buy her flowers (they're very inexpensive when you consider what rich dividends they pay!)

take her for candlelit suppers (in all surveys of 'what women consider romantic', dinner by candlelight scores very high).

Don't

ignore her all evening when you're out at a party together

fall in the door after work in the evening and forget to kiss her

flop down in front of the television and forget to talk to her all evening

wander around the bedroom in smelly socks

get into bed unshaven or unwashed

assume that once in bed, you can simply leap on her without any preliminaries

fall asleep the moment you've reached your climax (you could at least say 'Goodnight'!).

Romance, Emotion and Sexuality in Men

The outstanding US expert on sex, Dr Bernie Zilbergeld, neatly encapsulated an all-too-common male view of male sexuality and what man is supposed to contribute to the sex relationship in his famous phrase which describes a man's fantasy-view of his penis: 'two foot long, and hard as steel, and it goes all night...'

Of course, this phallic-orientated, male chauvinistic attitude is quite ridiculous! But most men will find echoes of it in the back of their own minds. And it's as well for women to bear in mind that this attitude exists – because it explains many of the stranger aspects of male sexual behaviour!

In particular, it explains why men are so often worried about their phalluses. Most males have worries such as:

is it big enough?

will I be able to get it erect?

how long will I be able to keep it up?

will I be able to get it up *again*?

So if you're a woman, keep in mind the fact that a man's attitude to sex and love is likely

ROMANCE

to be very genitally orientated.

And if you're a man, just consider whether it wouldn't be better to move away from these old macho ideas. Thank heavens, as we move into the last years of the twentieth century, there's an increasing trend towards the idea of what's been called 'the new man' – the man who's more concerned with being gentle and caring and sharing with his partner than with being obsessed with his own phallus.

But whether he's a 'new man' or the most ghastly of old-style 'macho men', the fact is that he too *probably needs a spot of romance in his love-life*. So I'll conclude this section with a few hints to help women make their partners feel romantic – and loved.

Romantic Tips for Women

Do:
tell him he's handsome – even if he isn't

take the trouble to see to your make-up and hair before you meet him (aggrieved feminists please note: I have given similar advice to *men* elsewhere in this book)

consider turning off the TV and giving him a cuddle instead.

Don't:
(as the song says) 'send him off with your hair all in curlers'

welcome him home with curlers in

wear terrible 'passion-killing' underwear in bed

heave a sigh of resignation as soon as you realize he has love-making in mind

say awful, unromantic things after love-making, like 'Would you please pass me a tissue to clear up this mess?'.

A Lifetime of Romance

Alas, today's fast-increasing trend is for marriages to go on the rocks. It seems to me that the best chance of reversing this alarming drift towards divorce is simply to *bring back romance*.

A ward sister recently told me about an old lady whom she had been nursing. This woman was 87 and had been married for about 60 years – yet before every visiting time she took enormous care to put on an elegant lace gown, make herself up beautifully, and dab a spot of perfume behind her ears.

Why? 'Well,' she told the ward sister, 'my husband is a *very* romantic man, you know...'

It gives you fresh hope, doesn't it?

RUBBING OILS

Rubbing Oils

The great US sex researchers Masters and Johnson found that the use of a massage oil was very helpful to couples with sexual difficulties. And of course, masseurs (and masseuses) have known for thousands of years that a body massage is improved by the use of an oil. You too may find a body oil helpful – to rub on the sexual or non-sexual parts of your partner's body, as you choose.

Important considerations are that the oil shouldn't be harmful or irritant to the skin or genitals; that it shouldn't stain the sheets!

Sex shops sell preparations with names like Love Oil, Love Cream, Joy Jelly, and Emotion Lotion! These usually contain perfumes, so there is a small risk of a sensitivity reaction if they are applied to delicate tissues.

In fact, vast numbers of couples in Britain, America and other countries have discovered that equally good results can be achieved by gently anointing each other's bodies with simple products such as baby oil or body lotion. For best results, remember to warm the oil in your hands before rubbing it into your loved one's shoulders, arms or whererever.

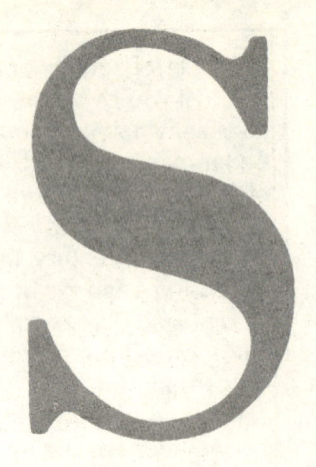

SETTLING DOWN • SEX DRIVE

Settling Down

Perhaps fortunately for the future of humanity, the great majority of women and men regard it as desirable to settle down with one partner for life, either in marriage or by living together.

Most couples – even those who have played the field for some years – are only too glad to settle into a mutual loving relationship in which they devote themselves to each other permanently – and have sex only with each other.

How often should they have sex? I wish I had a pound for every time somebody has written in asking me this question! The answer is that there are no very definite rules.

Dr Kinsey was the first to establish that the 'average' couple made love 2.4 times a week. At the beginning of 'settling down', couples tend to make love a little more often than this but later it's a little less. Other surveys over the last 40 years or so have confirmed that he was roughly right. But the important thing to realize is that as long as *both* partners are happy, it doesn't matter how often they make love.

The real problem arises when (as is so often the case) one partner wants to have sex frequently, while the other doesn't. This often happens, and when a woman who likes intercourse four times a week marries a man who only likes it once a month (or, indeed, *vice versa*), then trouble is brewing! Indeed, under these circumstances it's quite unusual for the marriage to survive. It is therefore important to try to marry somebody with more or less the same amount of interest in sex.

Q I am extremely passionate in mid-cycle, but then my sex drive vanishes. Round about ovulation, my sexual instincts are at full steam, and I lust after my husband.

Then after I've tired him out – that's it for the rest of the month. Can I do anything about this?

A Well, some women are like you. P'raps it's nature's way of ensuring that sex is most likely when you're at your most fertile.

However, two possibilities do occur to me. Firstly you may be losing interest in the second half of the cycle because of some sort of 'pre-menstrual syndrome'. If so,

SEX DRIVE • SEXUAL FANTASY

your doc might be willing to consider hormone treatment – e.g. with the dreaded progesterone suppositoires. And, second like some women, you may have a deeper feeling that sex should only be enjoyable when conception is possible. Psychotherpy could help this.

If neither of these suggestions is correct then just be happy that you're having a great time in the middle of the month.

Q My husband enjoys playing sex games during our love-making. If I say that I find them disgusting, he gets very upset and says it must be that I don't love him.

For instance, he wants to rub fruit-flavoured gel onto our bodies so that we can lick it off afterwards.

How can I get it through to him, without upsetting him, that these things are a turn off for me?

A Difficult, ma'am. People have wildly differing views on what is exciting, and what is disgusting in the bedroom.

My feeling is that you ought to be utterly frank and honest: write down a list of sex practices that you find repellent, hand it to him and say that – as much as you love him – you wouldn't want to do these with *anybody*.

If he takes that personally, then I'm afraid that's his problem.

Incidentally, re the 'fruit flavoured gel' which you find distasteful: it might just be worth trying fruit-flavoured 'Booby-Drops'. Since these are designer-made for love-making, they could be more aesthetically acceptable to you.

Q My husband wants to kiss my bottom intimately. Is this wise?

A No. Anilingus, or anilinctus, as it is also called, is thought to be responsible for the very high incidence of hepatitis in male homosexuals.

Q My fiancé wants me to use cocaine with him, and says it will improve our sexual satisfaction. What do you think?

A I think he's crazy. He'll probably end up impotent – and *you'll* probably end up in jail or in the cemetery (neither of which places is particularly noted for sexual satisfaction).

SEXUAL FANTASY

Q I would do almost anything sexually to keep my man, but now he's got this persistent kinky idea that he wants to urinate inside me.

A Well, don't let him! I get quite a few letters about various urinary games. Some are fairly harmless, but I reckon this one could damage your delicate vaginal tissues. Next time he asks, tell him to p...off.

Q My husband and I have always had a romantic desire to make love in the sea. But when we tried last summer we weren't able to manage it. I just couldn't seem to get him in. Why? Is it something to do with sea water?

A Yes, although making love in the briny sounds very romantic, it can be quite tricky – especially if there are sharks about!

More seriously, there are two basic problems. One is that you may be a bit tensed up, particularly if you're afraid that you might be spotted by someone on a passing pedalo.

Secondly, the sea does tend to instantly wash away the feminine 'love juices' which are so essential for an amatory encounter. (NB This is why mermaids are so unsuccessful in reproducing – or so I believe.)

Anyway, the answer to all this is to use a simple water-stable vaginal lubricant – the type you can buy without embarrassment at any British chemist's.

This year, pack a tube without fail. Happy holidays!

Q My boyfriend is heavily into books like *The Story of O* and the works of the Marquis de Sade. He's obsessed with wanting to stick objects up my backside. Now he wants me to get engaged. Do you think I should!

A No! Anyone who has the bad taste to read boring books like *The Story of O* (which, despite its prominent place on station bookstalls, is only marginally less tedious than the works of the Marquis de Sade) is really not worth getting engaged to.

As to his sexual proclivities, he's clearly a nut, and you would be well-advised to drop him. I should tell him what to do with his engagement ring. But watch out – in view of his tastes, he'll probably take you literally!

SEXUAL FANTASY

Q My husband has been reading a lot of sex manuals and has decided to buy me something called a 'clitoris stimulator' for my birthday. Could you please explain what on earth this is?

A Well ma'am, it's a device which is intended to do what it says – that is stimulate your clitoris. Basically it's a little ring which fits around the base of your man's penis. On top of the ring is a protuberance with various bumps or ridges on it.

The general idea is that these are supposed to rub against your clitoris while your bloke is making love to you. In practice, the device doesn't work very well, and can slip sideways and give you a nasty poke in the groin. Happy Birthday!

Q My husband likes me to go out in the evening wearing no knickers. How would you view this?

A By lying on the floor, I suppose! Seriously, this is an increasingly common habit among women – mainly for health reasons. Wearing no knickers may be a bit draughty, but it probably does help to protect you against thrush and other common vaginal problems.

Q I read the best-seller *Lace* by Shirley Conran, and was surprised by the scene in which the Arab prince puts a wriggling goldfish into the heroine's vagina, in order to stimulate her. What would really happen if one did this?

A I don't think it would be very nice – particularly for the goldfish. Honestly, I think authors just stick these scenes into novels to make a sensation (Shirley Conran certainly achieved worldwide publicity with *that* particular idea).

I've never encountered anybody who was daft enough to use a goldfish as a vibrator – and I hope I never do.

Q My boyfriend wants to make love to me in his whirlpool bath. Are there any gynaecological risks in this?

A Well, you could get pregnant. To be serious, the main risks of whirlpool baths arise if

SEXUAL FANTASY

they're used by a lot of people. Thus, public and hotel tubs have been incriminated in outbreaks of skin rashes and sore eyes. Also, in America some 14 members of a women's racquet-ball team went in a whirlpool bath together, and caught legionnaires disease.

Q My fiancé and I are going to the States later this year, and he is quite determined that on the flight we should join the 'Mile High Club'.

I understand that you 'join' it by making love in an aeroplane when it is more than a mile up.

I was a bit doubtful initially, but I must say it sounds quite exciting. However, could we get into trouble? And would the lack of air pressure do me any harm?

A This is definitely rather naughty behaviour, you know. However, the 'Mile High Club' does exist, and I am told that many of its members are airline staff, for obvious reasons.

But please bear in mind the practicalities. It is very difficult to make love on an aeroplane seat (or seats) unless the plane is virtually deserted. The alternative – which, I believe, is how many members of the Club qualified – is to make love in the loo. That sounds a teeny bit sordid to me – and also very cramped. (You could get yourself caught on the soap dispenser.)

Now I'm told that the airlines don't often prosecute anybody for engaging in this unusual form of 'in-flight entertainment.' But it would be awfully embarrassing if you were caught.

On the other hand, they can hardly chuck you out! And, to answer your final query, there are no physiological ill-effects associated with making love in the sky, no matter how high you go.

Q My wife wants to make love in a sauna. I suppose this is all a very romantic, but is it technically possible? Surely the wooden seats would be far too hot for a couple to lie down on?

A I'm sorry it's taken some time to answer your question, sir – but it has required a bit of research in Finland and elsewhere.

Love-making in the sauna is frowned on by the Finns (and, indeed, by Haringey Borough Council). But it is, in fact, technically possible, and quite often practised in Nordic lands.

You'll recall that in the traditional Finnish sauna there are usually three levels of benches (or *lauteet*). Apparently, the simplest method of

SEXUAL FANTASY

love-making is for the *nainen* (or female partner) to sit on the second level of *lauteet* facing forwards. The *mies* (or male partner) then stands on the tiled floor in front of her and embraces her – taking care not to get overheated in the *löyly* (or steam). What all this does to the *verenpaine* (or blood pressure), I do not know. But afterwards, they both go off for a cold shower – or else jump in the lake.

Q My husband invariably wants to make love to the sound of symphonic music. Is this unusual?

A Not at all, ma'am! In fact, I'd strongly recommend Brahm's First, Beethoven's Fifth, and Berlioz's *Fantastic*.

But think twice about Tchaikovsky's *Pathetique* and Schubert's *Unfinished*...

Q My husband read *Fear of Flying* by Erica Jong, in which the heroine brings another woman to a climax with a champagne bottle. Now he wants to do the same thing to me.

A A naff idea, ma'am. Very few things should be poked up the vagina, apart from the structure which nature, through some miricle, designed to fit it so perfectly.

Many couples who go in for these penetrative vaginal games don't realise that a woman's tissues are delicate, and tear easily.

Furthermore the magazine, *World Medicine* reported a case in which a Cumbrian couple tried to use a bottle of Bollinger as a dildo. Three months later, the cork had to be surgically removed...

Q My husband is always thinking up romantic and sexy things to do to me. But is his latest idea safe? He wants to bring home flowers, and use them to 'decorate' the various openings of my body.

A Well, if he only wants to stick a hibiscus blossom (*without* stem) in your ear, that's OK.

But pushing floral tributes up people's naughty bits is really not on! It can lead to infection, or damage delicate tissues.

Indeed, I remember a young bridegroom whom we had to operate on to remove the carnation stem which his 'stag night' pals had unwisely jammed into a very unfortunate place!

SEXUAL FANTASY • SEXUAL HARASSMENT

Sexual Fantasy

I'm always entertained by those mysterious small ads for 'rainwear' which appear in the most respectable newspapers. In case you don't know, these adverts are keenly perused by a very large number of people who – for some reason – are into making love with each other in plastic macs!

I suppose one shouldn't really make fun of other people's sexual habits. But I'm only poking *gentle* fun, especially as the 'rainwear lovers' do at least have the merit of being totally harmless to anyone else

Anyway, this month I'm intrigued to find out that worldwide there are now so many of them they've actually formed an international society, with its own quarterly journal, giving hints on rainwear fashions, plus details of barbecues, social evenings, and heaven knows what else.

It's called *La Société Mackintosh Internationale* (or if you're German, *Die Internationale Mackintosh Gesellschaft*).

If any readers are into that sort of thing, then as the *Société's* brochure says:

Pourquoi ne pas vous informer avec plus de détails . . . vous n'avez qu'à envoyer une enveloppe addressée à vous-même, avec un timbre postal, a l'addresse suivante: La Société Mackintosh Internationale, PO Box No 33, Horley, Surrey RH6 8NB.

Q My boyfriend wants to have intercourse with him while we are ice-skating. Is this really possible?

A Sounds chilly, and liable to get you arrested. But there are certain Torville-and-Dean-type poses in which it would be distinctly possible.

However, don't fall over – or you may discover a new definition of the word frigidity . . .

Q I am having a lot of trouble with two men in my office. They pinch my bottom and make offensive remarks about my breasts. Any suggestions?

A It's become increasingly clear in recent years that a lot of women are justifiably very upset by this tedious kind of sexual harassment at work.

127

SEXUAL HARASSMENT

Anyone who is subjected to attentions which she resents should consider these guidelines:

object *at once* – if you let things go on, they may get worse

if you belong to a union, complain at once – preferably to a female official

talk to other women at work about the problem

if necessary, tell the man that you'll complain to higher authority about his behaviour

if he *is* 'higher authority', then consider whether it's worth going to a lawyer – or the police.

if nothing can be done, don't stay in a job where you're miserable – leave

While I'm on the subject of sexual harassment at work, could I draw attention to one particularly dreadful manifestation of it?

Ever since I qualified in the early 60s, I've come across cases where lunatics working in factories have thought it a 'great joke' to put a high-pressure air hose up colleagues' skirts. *If the compressed air enters the victim's body (through the vagina or rectum), terrible damage can be done.*

Just before I wrote this book, yet another case of this form of harassment came before the courts. The woman victim escaped with her life, but was left with a permanent colostomy. I hope the man who did it is pleased with himself.

Q I am very surprised by what appears to be a new trend in sexual behaviour. These days, whenever we invite some couple over, the husband seems to go out of his way to catch me alone after dinner in the kitchen and grope me. Is this considered 'socially acceptable' today, or what?

A Well now you come to mention it, it does seem to me that these days the social after-dinner goodnight kiss has been widely replaced by the social after-dinner goodnight grope. All kinds of blokes, appear to think that if they're invited somewhere to dinner, this means that they're entitled to a bit of a cuddle with the hostess afterwards.

I suppose this doesn't matter very much if the hostess is keen on that sort of thing. But sexual harassment is *never* justifiable – even in the erotic post-prandial atmosphere so often induced by good food and good wine.

So cooks (of whichever sex) be careful whom you invite into the kitchen to help with the washing-up. If in doubt, hit'em with your wok.

THE TESTICLE

The Testicle

T

It is fairly important for a woman to have a working knowledge of the male testicle – if only because it's so awfully easy for her to damage it in bed!

All too commonly, a swiftly-raised feminine knee catches a chap in the wrong place, and immediately deprives him of the power of speech (not to mention anything else) for quite a while.

Happily, the pain and shock is as a rule only temporary, and I have not known any gent to suffer permanent harm or infertility as a result of such a bedtime accident.

But the testicle (also known as the testis, or 'ball'), is an incredibly pain sensitive part of the male body. This fact is vital to remember if you're attacked by a man. If at all possible, smash him as hard as you can in the testicles with knee, foot, fist, umbrella or whatever – and then run like hell, because (as I say) the disability is only temporary!

Turning to happier topics, the testicle is of course the source of the millions of sperms whose aim in life is to unite with a ripe ovum from your ovary and so form a baby.

The sperms which are produced by the testicle find their

THE TESTICLE

way up through a man's 'plumbing', in order to be ejaculated at the moment of climax. Anything up to 500 million of these crafty little rascals are produced in a single orgasm.

The two testicles have another function, which is to produce the male sex hormones, which give a lad his secondary male sex characteristics of hairiness muscularity, stroppiness, aggressive driving, and so on.

Each testicle is rather like a flattened ping-pong ball in shape and size. Average dimensions are about one and three quarter inches long, one and a quarter inches deep, and one inch thick.

Blokes are always worrying about the size of their testicles, but the actual dimensions matter little, provided the things work all right. If a man appears to be firing on both cylinders, then he needn't worry.

It's quite common for one testis to be slightly smaller than the other, and this too is quite normal. In virtually all men, one orb hangs slightly lower than the other but the reason for this is not known. A curious property of the testis is that it will retract rapidly upwards if it's threatened in any way. Try poking the inside of your man's thigh with a pencil and you'll see what I mean!

Testicles occasionally have to be removed because of accident or disease. Happily, these days it's possible to replace a lost testis with a plastic one which feels like the real thing.

Q If I refuse to let my fiancé make love to me, he complains that he gets an extremely intense pain in he testicles. Isn't he making all this up?

A Nope. If a bloke is sexually excited by kissing and cuddling but doesn't get the chance to reach a climax, he very often *does* get pain in his testicles.

This common ache is known as 'the gravels' or 'lover's nuts'. But my friend and colleague Dr Richard Gordon (remember *Doctor In The House?*) long ago christened it with the rather more elegant appellation of *orchitis amorosa acuta*.

Some women get a similar ache – possibly originating in their ovaries – when they've been stimulated but deprived of reaching an orgasm. So quite seriously, this 'frustration pain' is pretty widespread in both sexes.

The cure, I'm afraid, is still to come.

Troilism

This is an activity, common in some quarters, in which three people go to bed together. I make no moral comment on this, because that's not my brief. It's clear the troilism appeals to a lot of people for a variety of reasons. There are two types:

The Two Women in Bed with One Man Situation

This appeals to most males' sexual fantasies of course – since studies show that secretly, most men are very attracted by the idea of going to bed with as many women as possible – 50 or 100 perhaps. Girlie magazines encourage this sort of fantasy with the more girls the merrier, all of them eager to be satisfied! In reality, this wouldn't do the man a lot of good, since one man usually has enough trouble satisfying *one* woman – let alone two (or 100!).

It's also a little difficult to see what the two women are supposed to get out of this kind of troilism, unless, they have lesbian tendencies. My suspicion – based on talking to a number of people who've gone in for troilism – is that what the girls usually get out of it is *money*.

The Two Men in Bed with One Women Situation

As far as I can make out, this definitely does have an appeal for some women (though emphatically *not* for most) because of the higher chance of sexual satisfaction – and the feeling of being admired and wanted by not just one man, but two.

Why this situation appeals to some *men* isn't entirely clear. But there does seem to be a tendency for some men to feel their own sexual efforts to satisfy their partners aren't really sufficient, and should be augmented by those of good old Charlie down the road.

I have to say that I think there's a very real danger that if good old Charlie is any use in bed, he might end up going off with the woman (or, for all I know, with the other man!).

VAGINA • VAGINAL DRYNESS

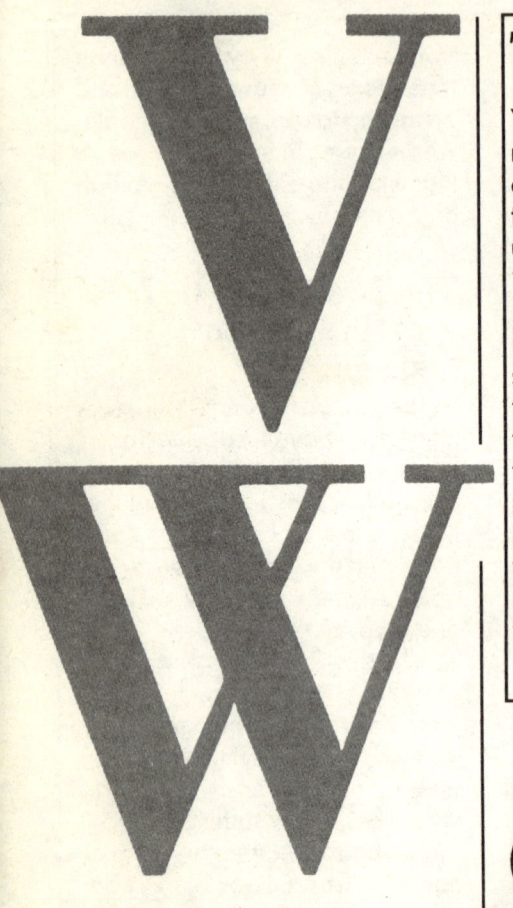

The Vagina

Your vagina is one of the most marvellously-designed structures on Earth. Yet the amazing thing is that so many women are brought up to believe that the vagina is 'nasty', 'dirty', or 'not nice'.

In fact, it's none of these things. It's a warm, pink, well-cushioned sheath which is perfect for its intended function in life. That function – let's not mince words – is to fit snugly and lovingly round the penis, so that the sperms are deposited in the right place, and so that both partners derive the maximum possible enjoyment from the act of love.

Regrettably, a lot of people

Q I am a 52-year-old woman. After many years of celibacy, I've started a wonderful relationship with a young man. The only problem is that I am distressingly sore and dry during lovemaking. Why?

A It's probably a minor hormone deficiency – common in the over-50s. To begin with, try using a lubricant such as KY Jelly or Durol –

VAGINA • VAGINAL DRYNESS

don't realize that the vagina is such a capacious and comfortably-upholstered channel. Instead they think it's a very tight passage, up which a man's penis can only be forced with difficulty and with pain.

This is nonsense. In reality, there's a vast amount of room inside the vagina. It 'balloons out' and lengthens quite dramatically during sexual excitement.

When you come to think of it, the vagina *has* to be a pretty distensible organ, because it must be able to dilate widely enough to let a baby's head through.

But, in addition to being remarkably distensible, it can also contract down, particularly at orgasm, to fit perfectly around the penis.

The other thing which the vagina can do is to produce the 'love juices' – the erotically-induced secretions which lubricate the movements of intercourse.

With their bizarre intra-vaginal camera, the US sex researchers Masters and Johnson have shown that when a woman becomes sexually aroused, it's the walls of her vagina which suddenly start pouring out the love juices.

All in all then, ladies, that's a beautiful and a marvellously efficient structure that you've got there.

---

buyable without embarrassment at any large chemist's. If that fails, ask your doc about hormone creams.

Q My first baby is now five months old. Since she was born, I have lost all my libido, and my vagina is very dry during lovemaking.

A This is very common, ma'am. The cause if probably to do with the sudden drop in hormones after a baby is born, though it could simply be due to lack of sleep or breastfeeding.

Unfortunately, we haven't come up with any very effective way of treating the lack of libido. But it *does* nearly always go away in the fullness of time. If not, go to a Family Planning Clinic for help.

Getting round the problem of vaginal dryness, however, is quite simple and a lubricant like Durol or KY would probably make life easier for both of you.

VAGINAL DRYNESS

Vaginal Dryness

I recently picked up a French women's magazine, whose cover bore a picture of a rather worried looking model, plus the caption '*Madame – avez-vous la SV?*'

Opening the mag, I rapidly found that the mysterious letters 'SV' stood for '*sécheresse vaginale*' – vaginal dryness.

Complaints of vaginal dryness are very common in the UK, France and doubtless most other countries in the world – because dryness makes it very difficult for a woman to have intercourse.

And even if she can just about manage it, it's likely to be at best unenjoyable, and at worst very sore and painful. (It often makes her bloke very red and sore too!)

So why does '*la SV*' occur?

Well, it's not usually due to any physical disorder, except in the case of women who've passed the menopause.

The latter do very often get distressing dryness, due to the fall in their female hormone levels. Happily, this can usually be put right by either: (a) taking female hormone tablets prescribed by a doc; or (b) using a female hormonal vaginal cream (also prescription only).

But among the rest of the female population, vaginal dryness isn't usually a disease or disorder or deficiency.

It's a failure of your 'love juice glands' to lubricate, for two possible reasons: (a) because your man hasn't stimulated you enough by love play; (b) because you're not relaxed enough.

Obviously, the two things often go together. Problem (a) can be overcome by insisting that your man learns and uses the basic techniques of foreplay. Problem (b) can be difficult, except where there is some clear-cut reason for your tension – for instance a recent episiotomy, or a recent vaginal infection.

Usually the best thing in severe cases is to see a woman doctor at a Family Planning Clinic for a spot of counselling plus vaginal relaxation exercises.

But in the many milder cases, things usually turn out OK if you use a bland vaginal lubricant for a while. KY Jelly is the traditional one, and another fluid one is called Senselle. Both can be bought cheaply over the counter, and you can apply them to your chap as well as yourself.

It used to be thought that the pill caused vaginal dryness, but this now seems unlikely.

VAGINAL DRYNESS • VAGINAL SLACKNESS

Q I am a very lucky girl with a loving, caring, desirable boyfriend. Only problem: I get so sore when we make love that we have to abandon it after a few minutes. Can you help? My boyfriend is not unduly large. And I don't think it's a 'love juice' problem.

A Well, I rather suspect it is, and I think things will get better over the years as you relax – and produce more juices.

But in the meantime, you should go to any chemist and buy a lubricant which will 'ease the passage'.

If they don't work, you and your chap should go to a Family Planning Clinic for technical advice.

Q My vagina is now so loose that I thought my husband would seek sex elsewhere. In order to tighten things up, I have been putting a tampon up my bottom before sex. Is this wise?

A I don't think it's a good idea, ma'am. Sorry to hear about your problems, but I suggest you see a gynaecologist to discuss a tightening up operation.

Vaginal Slackness

So many readers have written in asking where they could buy devices which help improve women's pelvic muscle tone, when the vagina has become slack after having children that I thought I'd better print full details. Perhaps one of the following would make a nice Christmas present!

Anyway, the most sensible vaginal muscle developer seems to me to be the 'Femtone', which is available for £15 (including p & p) from Aleph One Ltd, *The Old Courthouse, Bottisham, Cambridgeshire CB5 9BA*.

The same firm also supply the extraordinary biofeedback perineometer (!), which enables you to play back you vaginal contractions on a loudspeaker, if you fancy that sort of thing! But it does cost a hefty 500 quid!

An alternative is to buy the naughty 'Geisha Balls' or 'Duo Balls'. They are available at any sex shop for a few pounds, and can be 'worn' all day.

Those who use them to develop their vagina muscles say that they're *wickedly* agreeable to use – but they do tend to produce a loud 'clonking' sound as you walk about, which may be a mite embarrassing . . .

VAGINAL SLACKNESS

Flexing Your Vaginal Muscles

The vaginal muscles form the front part of the pelvic floor muscles – which make up a sort of 'diaphragm' stretched across the lower part of your body.

Now these muscles make a ring round the opening of your vagina, so that they gently grip your man's penis when you are making love with him.

Unfortunately, in quite a lot of women these vaginal muscles go into an involuntary spasm whenever any approach is made to their vaginas. This is the all-to-common condition of 'vaginismus', which makes intercourse painful or down-right impossible.

It is claimed that violent spasm of these vaginal muscles is the cause of rare cases of *penis captivus*. This is the alleged syndrome in which the man becomes trapped inside the woman and cannot withdraw.

Anyway, how do you flex your vaginal muscles?

Quite simple, really. Next time you are making love, just 'twitch' the lower front part of your body, as if you were trying to stop yourself from spending a penny.

Your man will immediately feel a gentle but pleasant squeezing sensation. Indeed, it may be that as a result he will immediately reach an unwanted early climax, and spend the rest of the evening cursing me! So perhaps you'd better warn him first.

What I have described is actually the first of the two 'Kegel exercises', which strengthen a woman's muscles, and help her to avoid prolapse in later life.

You can also use the second Kegel exercise during lovemaking. This involves tightening up the muscles a little further back (again, with a bit of a 'twitch') as if you were trying to prevent a bowel action. This also produces a gentle vaginal squeeze – which may be perceived by the man as being a little deeper inside.

There are those who claim that after months of practice on these two exercises, a determined woman can acquire such yoga-like control of her vagina muscles that she can use the outer and inner muscles alternately.

If this is true (and it may be so), she would presumably emulate the young lady of Brussels –

Whose pride was her vaginal muscles;
She could easily plex them,
And so interfex them
As to whistle love songs through her bustles!

VAGINAL SORENESS

Q We are 20 lovely and loving ladies from Farnham, Surrey, and we disagree with your theory about penis size and vaginal soreness.

You said that the woman who thought her boyfriend's penis was too large for her (because she could not have sex with him) was probably wrong – and just suffering from *vaginismus* (vaginal muscle spasm).

Well, some of the 20 ladies in our office have had experiences similar to that described in the reader's letter. And in no case had it anything to do with *vaginismus*, since everything was OK with subsequent partners. You clearly are misinformed!

A Dear lovely (and loving) ladies: we are slightly at cross-purposes here.

Most women have had the experience of being unable to make love with a particular bloke because of one or more of the following factors:

he was too clumsy

he tried to get in before she was ready

she was tensed up

she had some painful vaginal infection (such as thrush)

she'd recently had an episiotomy, or a birth-tear, stitched up

All of these factors are liable to cause intense pain. And quite understandably, that pain frequently produces a terrific 'tightening up' of the vaginal muscles. *That is how* vaginismus *begins.*

With tenderness and commonsense on the part of both partners, the vaginal spasm should go away quite soon – though occasionally it takes months or years.

I repeat that is very, very rare for a couple to find that the man's penis is so big that it genuinely will not go into the vagina.

PS Sorry I had to cut your letter down. It was too long to fit in (if you'll forgive the phrase)!

Q Recently I met a man whom I would like to marry. But the first time we made love left me with considerable soreness next day. And on the next occasion, it was quite impossible.

Since then, a friend has told me that some couples simply cannot make love because the man's penis is too big or the wrong shape. Is this right?

A Such cases are so very, rare that I've never seen one in my life.

What's far more likely is this. You

137

VAGINAL WIND • VAGINISMUS

were able to achieve intercourse the first time, but (for some reason which a doctor would need to sort out) this caused soreness the following day.

Such soreness is often the trigger for the very common condition called **vaginismus** (vaginal muscle spasm) The pain tends to make intercourse difficult or impossible.

So what you need to do now is to go along to an experienced woman doctor at a Family Planning Clinic. She'll examine you and (I hope) teach you the simple techniques of relaxation which will enable you to have painless love-making with your man.

Q I'm a girl in my late teens and my very embarrassing problem is (as my friends so delicately phrase it) 'fanny farting'!

Please don't laugh at me. I have only had intercourse with one partner in the past, and I found that when his penis was thrust into my vagina, it seemed to drive in air, compress it, and then push it out, so creating this ghastly noise.

I feel quite anxious about it at the moment, because of the fact that a new, close relationship with a man looks as though it's shortly going to become enhanced into a physical one (Hopefully!).

PS I think your column is ace!

Vaginismus

PAINFUL intercourse (and even complete inability to have intercourse) is frequently caused by vaginismus.

This is a disabling, involuntary spasm of the muscles which form a ring round the vagina, and comes on whenever a woman is sexually approached.

So if you suffer from vaginismus, you'll doubtless have found that if a man tries to make love to you, the muscles of your vagina close in, like a mouth saying 'No' – and also that your thigh and tummy muscles tend to tighten up at the same time, to protect your vaginal area.

If you have vaginismus quite badly, then you won't even be able to tolerate petting – because your body will tense and curl up self-protectively as soon as a man puts his hand anywhere near your thighs.

A Thank you so much – us gents do always appreciate complimentary remarks about our columns.

Now let's be quite serious about this problem of 'vaginal wind'. Long ago, I wrote about this com-

VAGINAL WIND • VAGINISMUS

In a minority of cases, it's sparked off by some painful vaginal condition – like a bad attack of thrush, or an extremely tender episiotomy scar (caused by stitches after childbirth). An attempt at intercourse leads to intense pain; this produces muscle spasm which continues for some months. Because of the spasm, the next attempt causes more pain – and so on.

But in most women with vaginismus, there isn't a physical cause. The difficulty is an emotional one though its not intentional (something which men find very difficult to understand!). You see, even today, large numbers of women grow up with the belief that any kind of penetration of the vagina is very dangerous. Characteristically, they are terrified of using tampons. They also react very evasively or angrily if a doctor wants to do a vaginal examination. (Quite often, the doc makes the big mistake of reacting angrily too – and this may foul up their relationship.)

So, a woman who has vaginismus will have great difficulty in relaxing sufficiently to allow intercourse. She may even be a 'virgin wife'.

Happily, women doctors – mostly working in Family Planning Clinics – have developed a form of psychotherapy (Combined with yoga-like exercises) which enables a vaginismal woman to gain control over her muscles. Countless, women have had their sex lives revolutionised through this method. If you have problems with vaginismus, ask your local Family Planning Clinic if they have a woman doctor practising this form of therapy. If they haven't then write (enclosing sae) to the Institute of Psychosexual Medicine, *11 Chandos St, London W1M 9DE.*

mon difficulty in **SHE**. In my lofty medical arrogance, I declared that it only affected women whose vaginas were too lax because of child-bearing.

How wrong I was! I was nearly blown away by a great blast of letters from women who had no babies at all – but were plagued by the same noisome problem.

I've often told that story at medical meetings – just to show how wrong us docs can be. But unfortunately, *at none of these meetings has any doctor been able to suggest a cure for this vaginal flatulence.*

The best I can suggest is that you

VAS DEFERENS • VASECTOMY

use a vaginal aerosol-foam contraceptive, such as Emko or Delfen (no relation!), to try and 'soak up' the air which has been forced into your vagina.

But what if this doesn't work? Well, just bear in mind that it takes *two* to cause this compression of air; in other words, it's the bloke's problem as well as yours, because he's the one that's pushing it in!

So if it happens with your new lover (and it may not), just say 'Ooops – you've driven some air into me with that great piston of yours!'

If he doesnt laugh at *that*, he's probably not worth going to bed with.

Q My husband is thinking of having a vasectomy, but what we do not understand is this: would he still produce the fluid after the operation?

A Vasectomy has become fantastically popular this last year or so – a fact which has enabled many a surgeon to re-furnish the

---

The Vas Deferens

Here's an important organ which is not very well known to the public. It's the vas deferens – more commonly referred to as 'the vas' (usually pronounced 'vass', rhyming with 'lass'). 'Vas' is Latin for 'vessel', and 'deferens' means 'bringing'. And the vas deferens is the tube which brings sperm up from the testicle towards the penis.

A man normally has two of these tubes; a few men have three, but this is not an advantage to them as we shall see. The vas looks very like a thin piece of spaghetti. It can be felt with the fingertips through the skin of a man's scrotum as it runs up towards the groin.

The reason why there is such a lot of interest in the vas these days is that *it is the bit that is cut in a vasectomy*. Vasectomy just means 'cutting through the vas'.

This popular operation (well over a hundred thousand are being done world-wide every year) just involves making two tiny incisions in the skin of the scrotum, working through them to cut through each vas and tying the ends.

Why are men who have a *third* vas at a disadvantage? Because the surgeon probably will not realize they have an extra vas

VIBRATORS

front room. Lots of couples ask this question – and the answer is that the man *does* continue to produce fluid in exactly the same way as before at his climax. This is because the sperms are so tiny that their absence makes practically no difference at all to its volume.

Q **I am embarrassed to say that because my husband's love-making does not entirely satisfy me, I usually bring myself to a climax afterwards with a vibrator.**

deferens, and will fail to cut it. In such cases, the vasectomy won't work! However, the sperm test which is done a couple of months or so after a vasectomy will detect the fact that there is another vas deferens, still sending up vast supplies of spermatozoa. The third vas can them be cut and tied off too.

The vas deferens does *not* seem to have any hormonal function. So, cutting through it dosen't interfere with a man's production of sex hormones, or with his virility. It just gives him a great feeling of coinfidence that he is no longer exposing his female partner to the risk of unwanted pregnancy.

My problem is this. We're going abroad on a business trip soon, and I wonder if I could get into difficulties if the customs found the device in my luggage?

A Within Western Europe and North America, customs officers have been fairly used to vibrators. But you might risk confiscation and public embarrassment if you tried to import one into certain Middle Eastern countries. Also, I suggest you take the batteries out: I've heard of one going off in a plane and causing a bomb alert.

Q **Much to my alarm, I have found that recently my wife has been doing something rather unusual at the end of intercourse. After I have 'finished' she produces a vibrator and used it to bring herself to her climax. Is this abnormal?**

A Well sir, it's increasingly common these days. Most women do *not* regularly reach a climax during intercourse. I don't think it's unreasonable for a woman who is still unsatisfied after her man's orgasm to decide to take matters into her own hands (so to speak).

Not all men can cope with this recent trend in female sexuality. But

VIBRATORS

I think you should curb your 'alarm' – and just be glad that your missus has found a way of giving herself a buzz...

Q **I have decided that it would be fun to buy a vibrator for me and my husband to use. But I really don't want to go in one of those dreadful sex shops, so where could I get one?**

A Many readers will throw up their hands in horror at the idea of a woman wanting to buy a vibrator. When these devices first came on to the market, I used to think they be blunt – not all that skilled at, or enthusiastic about, love-play.

In addition, quite a lot of couples just use vibrators for sheer fun – or perhaps to spare them a lot of effort when they're tired. (One woman told me quite frankly that when her husband was exhausted, they were both more than happy for her to 'finish herself off' with a vibrator.)

The usual thing is for one or other partner just to hold them gently near or on the woman's clitoris, and let the gentle 'buzzing' motion have its effect.

As you'll discover, some vibrators are actually penis-shaped, and can be placed in the vagina. I suspect that these were invented by men; they certainly don't seem to be as popular with women as the clitoral vibrators.

If you do decide to put a vibrator inside the vagina, you should:

Vibrators

Vibrators have been the one really big success of the sex aid industry. Much to my initial surprise, I've had many letters from women who have found them useful in overcoming lack of libido and failure to reach a climax.

The very idea of a vibrator puts many people off to begin with. But a considerable number of patients actually discover that they like them. They seem to be particularly helpful to three groups of females:

women who are on their own (either temporarily or permanently)

women whose husbands are unable to stimulate them properly because of disability (e.g. arthritis)

women whose partners are – to

VIBRATORS

were quite crazy – but eventually I realised that a vast number of women (and some men) do find them fun to use in bed. They can also be helpful for sexual problems.

Now, I quite understand your reluctance to visit some sleazy sex shop to buy a vibrator – but you don't have to these days.

Perfectly reputable chain stores do now sell 'electrical massagers' or 'beauty massagers' which work admirably as vibrators. My researchers indicate that many women buy them without embarrassment as 'beauty aids'.

For instance, the Clairol Beauty Massage system (around £9.95 at large chemists) can be used successfully to put a little extra voltage

---

make absolutely sure that the device is clean

make certain that there are no rough or jagged bits which could hurt

insert *very* gently, perhaps using a lubricant.

Most vibrators are battery-powered, but there are also mains-powered, vibrators. Interestingly these devices are now sold on a massive scale all over the western world in pharmacies and electrical goods shops (rather than sex shops) as 'massagers'.

Ostensibly, they are supposed to be either for 'beauty' or for 'rheumatism' – take your pick! – but it's well known that a vast number of women use the mains-powered massagers for sexual pleasure or relief.

Finally, two words of warning about vibrators – one serious

and one not so serious. Firstly, there's a disturbing tendency nowadays to use vibrators rectally, for added sensual stimulation. Indeed, some brands are actually *sold* as 'rectal vibrators' (they're a lot thinner than the ordinary kind).

Using rectal vibrators is absolute madness. Quite apart from the hygiene problem mentioned in earlier chapters, there's the all-important fact that a vibrator can disappear up your bottom, never to be seen again! Or – to be more precise – it *will* be seen again, after a surgeon has operated on you to remove it.

The less serious point is this. Before you buy a vibrator, you should appreciate that virtually all these devices are very noisy! If you live with your in-laws or in an apartment with thin walls, then most probably a vibrator is *not* for you.

VIRGINITY • WIFE SWAPPING

into your love life. But in fact, nowadays you don't need to visit a shop to buy a 'vibe'.

In most liberated women's magazines, there are small ads indicating where you can purchase vibrators via mail order (or, perhaps one should say, female order...).

Q I am 25 years old and still a virgin. Personally, I would like to remain like this for quite a while, but people keep suggesting there's something wrong with me because I haven't had sex. What do you think?

A Old Delvin, him say: 'Good for you'! I dislike efforts to make people 'conform' sexually. I think there's far too much pressure put on women to lose their virginity these days, particularly by blokes who use lines like: 'You must be lesbian if you don't want to have intercourse.'

So hang on to your virginity if you want to. Obviously, you'll miss out on some fun, but I have to admit you'll miss out on a lot of monthly anxiety too.

Wife-swapping

Everything I've said about the dangers of open marriage applies with even more force to wife-swapping. This practice is now endemic in the relatively affluent suburbs of cities in the USA, Britain and Australia.

What usually happens is that a couple advertise in a 'contact magazine', and then selects a husband and wife from the replies they get – and I gather they get many.

They then meet up in a pub or bar, and see if they like the look of each other. If they do, they simply swap partners for the night.

The risks involved – particularly that of VD – are considerable. By going in for this kind of thing, you also put yourself in jeopardy of blackmail. A small number of couples who have indulged in it have been horrified to find their names splashed over the racier newspapers.

All of this makes it *very* dangerous living indeed (like 'feasting with panthers', as Oscar Wilde used to say in a different context).

Sexual Health and Well-being

AIDS

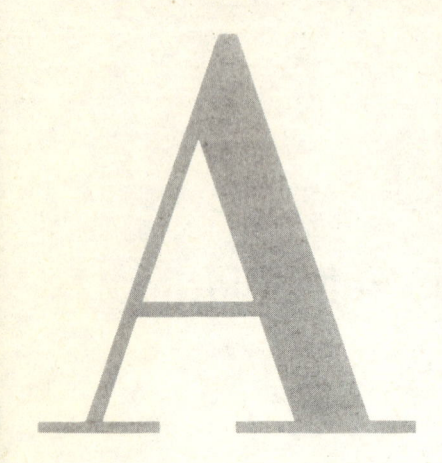

Q I'm a cabbie, and some people have the disgusting habit of holding banknotes in their mouths for a moment before they pay me. Is it possible for me to get AIDS from this?

A Well, I do agree that putting money in the mouth is a pretty mucky habit! (Talk about 'filthy lucre!').

But it would be very difficult to catch anything by accepting such a damp banknote – unless you promptly stuck it in your own mouth. Even then, I must stress that it still has not been proved that AIDS can be transmitted by saliva.

Q I have been warned against 'rimming' with my fiancé, because of the risk of AIDS.

But what actually *is* 'rimming'?

A Well, I'm afraid that 'rimming' is the exceedingly common practice of kissing and licking each other's bottoms.

Quite honestly, this practice *can't* be recommended hygiene-wise due to the fact that your *derrière* isn't exactly the cleanest part of your anatomy.

'Rimming' could give the two of

AIDS

you tummy upsets, or worse, worms.

Of course, you could catch AIDS from it if your fiancé were himself carrying the HIV virus, but rather more likely is that one of you might be a carrier of hepatitis, and might pass it on in this way. So all in all, I reckon this is a bum practice. Sorry.

Q Is there any danger of catching AIDS from the water in swimming pools?

Some people pass urine while they're swimming, so presumably this might infect the water.

A Some folk do indeed have the unfortunate habit of having a pee in swimming pools.

A swimming bath technician told me that chemical tests indicate that a substantial proportion of bathers do have this rather anti-social tendency. But don't worry; the chlorine in the water gets rid of most germs — including AIDS, I hope. Nonetheless, on aesthetic grounds I would try to avoid swallowing the water from any swimming pool, anywhere!

Q I was very worried by your comments in SHE about anal sex passing on AIDS. My husband and I do this sometimes. We have never had sex with anyone else. Are we in danger of AIDS?

A No. I've had several letters about this from worried readers. Although rectal sex is the most 'efficient' way of transmitting the AIDS virus, obviously this *can't* happen unless one of you already has it.

Q I have recently been on holiday to Central Africa and had an affair there.

I am awfully worried that this might have given me AIDS. How can I find out, without arousing my husband's suspicion?

A Well, I can't deny that you have some reason for concern, ma'am.

On the latest figures which I have available, only about 400 British women have developed AIDS after acquiring the HIV virus through intercourse.

But the majority of those caught the virus abroad — with Africa the most dangerous place of all.

So Central Africa is no place to have an affair these days! However, the odds against infection are still in your favour, and not all doctors would feel that you

AIDS

need subject yourself to the worry of having an HIV blood test.

Best move would be to go to the nearest large Genito-Urinary ('Special') Clinic for confidential counselling.

You live in London, and such clinics are located in all the London teaching hospitals. (You don't need a GP's letter.) Good luck.

Q I slept with a man at a party last week. What are the chances that he might have given me the HIV virus?

A At least 500 to one against at the moment — unless he was a bisexual, a drug addict, or from Central Africa or New York.

But please bear in mind that casual mating at parties is very much more likely to bring you certain other kinds of pelvic infection, such as chlamydia or gonorrhoea.

Furthermore, as we move into those 'nervous 90s' the risks of getting HIV from casual sexual dalliance will become much, much more frightening.

Q I'm a married man, but gay. I am terribly worried that I might give my wife an infection like AIDS, and I would like a check-up to set my mind at ease.

But I can't face the idea of going to one of those VD clinics and explaining to them that I am homosexual, or (I suppose) really bisexual.

A Well sir, let me reassure you that you certainly shouldn't encounter any prejudice at a clinic. What you probably don't realise is that quite a lot of clinic staff are likely to be gay themselves!

And I'm sure that, if you think about it, you'll see that there are perfectly understandable and praiseworthy reasons why they should have taken up this kind of work.

In view of your very worried state of mind, you shouldn't hesitate to go to the nearest Genito-Urinary ('Special') Clinic. They certainly won't bat an eyelid when you tell them you're AC/DC.

Q I've found out — to my great sadness — that my husband has been with a prostitute. Could this give me AIDS?

A The odds are still against it, but the risk of *other* forms of venereal infection (eg gonorrhoea) is fairly high. So it'd be best if both you and your husband went to a

AIDS

Genito-Urinary ('Special') Clinic for a confidential check-up.

The fact remains that prostitutes, many of whom are drug addicts, will almost certainly soon become an important source of AIDS virus, through sharing infected needles.

Indeed, it is believed that at least one British male may have already developed AIDS through going with prostitutes, although he might have acquired the virus through sharing a razor with friends who are heroin users.

Q My mother is at home dying of cancer, and I am having to sell my body to raise the money to look after her. So I need your advice: where I can go for health checks, especially for AIDS?

A If your letter is genuine, the situation you describe is absolutely terrible. You can get special help for your mother if you ring up the Medical Social Worker at the hospital where she has been treated, and ask her to make an application to the National Society for Cancer Relief.

I'm afraid you're quite right in thinking that prostitution greatly increases your risk of catching infections – including AIDS. You can get health checks – and that includes AIDS testing if necessary – from any of the 'Special Clinics' or 'Genito-Urinary Clinics' scattered across the country. Just ring the nearest large hospital and ask for the place and time of the next 'G-U Clinic.' Good luck.

Q My husband and I have a very good friend who is gay. I have quite often kissed him goodbye after a dinner party. Is there any danger I might have contracted AIDS?

A None whatever! With no disrespect to you, ma'am, I really am fed up with all this national panic about AIDS – and especially the way that certain people in the media have used it to vent their prejudices against gays.

I see that people have started doing crazy things like excluding gay blokes from pubs and clubs. That's bonkers! For a start, the odds against the average non-promiscuous gay having the disease are at least a thousand to one, by my calculations.

Furthermore, you *cannot* get the infection by being in the same pub, club, office, railway carriage or whatever with an infected person. All the evidence points to the fact that *very* intimate physical contact (usually actual intercourse) seems to be necessary in nearly all cases.

AIDS

I've had a number of letters from gay people who are worried about the disease. And I can assure you, I didn't disappear in a puff of blue smoke when I handled their notepaper!

I'd advise any gay person who's anxious about AIDS to ring the organisation called Gay Switchboard at 01-837 7324. They are receiving around 500 calls a week about AIDS at present, and they have sensible, up-to-the-minute advice about how to avoid this disease.

Q In the mid-1980s, I had an affair with a very nice guy. It ended amicably when I got engaged to someone else. But I got an awful fright last week when I heard by chance that this former lover has been known to have homosexual leanings. Is there any chance that he could have given me AIDS?

A I'm afraid that this is a situation in which more and more women are going to find themselves over the next few years. The number of bisexual blokes around is quite incredible! So before sleeping with a man, the woman of the Nervous Nineties would do well to ask herself: 'Has my feller ever been interested in *other* fellers?'

However, in your case I don't think you've got much to worry about. I say that for two reasons:

First, at the time years ago when you slept with this bisexual chap, there had only been about 100 cases of AIDS in the country.

Second, transmission of the virus is much less likely by the vaginal route than by the rectal one.

So provided you stuck to the orthodox way of making love, it's pretty unlikely that you've acquired AIDS from this guy.

Q I have slept around quite a bit in my life. And, quite frankly, I've enjoyed it! I've slept with one or two men who probably were a bit bisexual.

Do you think the AIDS outbreak should make me put a stop to my present lifestyle?

A I fear so – agreeable though you may have found it.

Certainly, no woman in this country should ever again have an affair with a man whom she suspects is 'AC/DC'.

Sleeping with 'straight' (heterosexual) males will probably remain *relatively* free of risk of AIDS till well into the 1990s – the decade which I've christened 'the Nervous Nineties'.

By that time, AIDS will almost

AIDS

certainly have hit the UK like a mediaeval plague.

Unless some miracle (like a vaccine) saves us, we're going to see death and social disruption on a scale which I find horrific to contemplate.

Q I was unfaithful to my husband three years ago, and now I have symptoms which I fear might be due to AIDS. Is this possible?

A Very unlikely, ma'am, I'm glad to say. I keep getting letters from women who are afraid that they've picked up AIDS. But I'd like to point out to all of you that at the time of writing, the total number of women in the entire country who have developed AIDS is only 150.

Sadly, this total will increase dramatically as we progress through this decade (which, sexually speaking, will be 'the Nervous Nineties', I'm afraid).

However, at the moment the chance of a brief affair giving a woman AIDS is just about nil. But if you have symptoms which worry you, then you can go to the nearest Genito-Urinary Clinic ('Special Clinic') and have free and confidential advice.

Q Is it possible for a woman to catch AIDS from having sexual intercourse with a man?

A Yes, it's possible. But it's now clear that rectal intercourse is a far more 'efficient' way of transmitting the virus. That's why about 80% of British cases so far have been male gays.

Ordinary sexual intercourse with a bloke *could* give you the germ – if he was infected with it – but you might be OK.

In practice, heterosexual intercourse with chaps will remain a very low-risk pastime for several years in the UK. But I feel that by the middle of the 1990s, there'll be so many AIDS cases around that a woman will have to think very, very carefully before agreeing to go to bed with her date.

Q I'm a gay male, and am terrified of AIDS. Where can I get some reliable information about it?

A Excellent – and frank – information leaflets are produced by the praiseworthy self-help organisation, the Terrence Higgins Trust. Send a large s.a.e. to them at *BM AIDS, London, WC1N 3XX*.

AIDS

Q If a husband has been unfaithful, do you think the wife should these days demand an HIV test before taking him back?

A Well, at the moment the chances of catching HIV from a heterosexual affair in this country are still low. That will start changing now that we've entered what I christened 'the nervous 90s'.

But the current situation is that unless your husband's adultery was with a 'high risk' woman, such as a drug addict, or somebody from one of the danger areas of the world (New York, Central and East Africa — and Edinburgh and Milan), it's many hundreds to one against him having HIV. So I don't think that a test should be the most important consideration in deciding whether to take him back.

Q I was appalled by your condemnation of rectal sex. My husband and I have always found this bedtime activity very intimate and soothing, particularly when I have a period and don't want vaginal intercourse.

As we do not have AIDS, surely there is no harm in it?

A Well ma'am, I seem to have upset quite a lot of readers who occasionally go in for this practice. (In fact, 40% of women who replied to the recent SHE sex survey said they had tried it.)

Rectal intercourse between a man and woman is illegal in England and Wales — though *not* illegal for two men over 21!

There's only a risk of AIDS if one partner has the virus but there are other hygiene risks from rectal sex. Hepatitis and viral warts can be passed on, so too can an odd infection known as 'the Gay Bowel Syndrome', I kid you not!

The common practice of oral-anal contact (rimming) can transmit a form of food poisoning called giordiasis — and just possibly amoebic dysentery too.

Naturally, if neither of you are carrying these infections, then you can't transmit them.

But a word of warning: it's often common for a woman to develop a vaginal discharge if she has rectal intercourse *followed* by vaginal intercourse.

Anything that has touched bottom must *not* then be inserted into the vagina — or at least without careful washing first.

AIDS

Q I am worried about getting bitten by mosquitoes when I go on holiday. Could they carry AIDS? I believe you said in SHE this was impossible. How do you know?

A I didn't say that at all! I too am a bit worried that mosquitoes which bite people who carry the AIDS virus are said to ingest the virus as they suck the person's blood.

Theoretically, it seems possible to me that a 'mozzie' could pass the virus on to the next person she bites — just as happens with malaria and yellow fever.

However, at the moment AIDS experts seem to think that this doesn't happen. The main reason why they say this is the fact that although AIDS is rampaging in Africa, very few African children have got it, thank heavens. Yet they are of course being bitten by mozzies all the time.

So, all in all, I reckon that an unwise holiday romance would be far, far more dangerous for you than a mosquito bite.

Q I have been married to my husband for 20 years, and seven years ago we went through a 'bad patch'. During that time, I am ashamed to say that I had an affair with my sister's husband. This was his only 'unfaithfulness' too.

Fortunately, we both came to our senses, and put it all behind us. I am now in love with my husband all over again.

But I am terrified that God will punish me by giving me AIDS. I am desperately upset and am losing weight fast. Could this affair have given me the virus?

A I'd say that it's virtually impossible that you could have caught AIDS from this affair, ma'am.

Your weight loss is almost certainly due to *depression*, and I beg you to see your doc and ask for help and treatment.

Actually, your letter is just one of many which I've received from women who are frightened that they may have picked up AIDS from a heterosexual affair.

I'd like to say to all of you that *if the affair was before 1985,* then it's at least a million to one against it having given you AIDS.

However *recent* heterosexual affairs are of course likely to be a bit more risky — because the AIDS virus is now so much more common.

Nevertheless, my rough calculation (based on the best figures currently available) suggests that *less than one in 200 of the sexually*

AIDS

active population is carrying the virus. And most of those are gay blokes.

So though the risk to women is gradually increasing, it's still quite small – except in those towns with high drug-abuse and prostitution rates, which are becoming notorious for AIDS.

Q I am a lesbian, and I wonder if it is safe for me to give blood, in view of the current AIDS scare?

A Perfectly OK. Lesbians are *not* particularly liable to AIDS – indeed, most kinds of sexual infection are rare among female homosexuals.

It's male gays who are specially liable to AIDS, particularly if they have been promiscuous in the past. Indeed, in view of recent tragedies in Australia and here – in which a number of babies and adults died after receiving blood from homosexual men – all gay males are now discouraged from giving blood.

Aids and Haemophiliacs

Re Aids and haemophilia: I've had several very worried enquiries from women whose fellers are haemophilia sufferers.

The AIDS situation for haemophiliacs and their sex partners is now very disturbing.

Haemophilia is (as most people know) the 'bleeding' disease – caused by a deficiency of a blood component called Factor VIII.

Nowadays, this vital factor can be extracted from donated blood, and given to haemophiliacs by injection so that the blood clots properly.

But thanks to a piece of what seems to me to have been unbelievable idiocy, Britain carried on importing most of its Factor VIII from America *long after the AIDS outbreak had started there.*

As a result, it is clear that over a quarter of the haemophiliacs in Britain have been infected with HIV virus.

Many of these are children, unfortunately. Others are adult males – and some of those have already infected their wives or girlfriends with the virus.

If your man is a haemophiliac, what you need to do is to join The Haemophilia Society (*PO Box 9, 16 Trinity Street, London, SE1 1DE*),

AIDS

and get their leaflet *Advice on Safer Sex*.

This clear and very frank pamphlet advises that you stick to the following sex rules:

Always use a sheath;
Always use *some other contraception as well* (because pregnancy MUST be avoided till you're completely certain that neither you nor your partner has the virus);
Avoid anal sex;
Don't share a toothbrush or razor (because it may transfer blood via cuts or gum abrasions).

ARTIFICIAL INSEMINATION

Q The doctors have advised my husband and me that we should use AIH (artificial insemination by husband) in order to conceive. But the NHS waiting list is a year long. Could we get it done privately?

A Yes, ma'am. For instance, the charity BPAS (HQ phone number Henley-in-Arden 3225) arranges AIH. They'll also advise you about a simple DIY kit which you could use at home.

Artificial Insemination

Artificial insemination is technically very easy to carry out, and has helped many couples to have much-wanted children. There are two types: AIH and Donor Insemination. In both cases the doctor simply takes some seminal fluid and injects it into the upper part of the woman's vagina at about the time of ovulation.

AIH

This means 'artificial insemination by the husband'. It's done in a few cases of premature ejaculation, and also when the husband has some anatomical abnormality which makes effective intercourse impossible.

Donor Insemination (still often known as 'AID')

This is used when the husband is completely infertile. Naturally, both husband and wife have to be completely happy that they will be able to accept a baby which was really fathered by another man.

It's also important to realise that Donor Insemination is far more contentious than AIH. It's illegal in some countries, and in *all* countries there may be legal problems about registering the parents' names on the child's birth certificate. Relatives and friends may not be too understanding, so most AID couples keep quiet about it.

In general, what happens is that the doctors or clinic who are providing the service have a list of donors — who are frequently medical students. Obviously, the chosen donor should roughly match the husband in general colouring, race and physical size. You will have to rely on the doctor or clinic for this —

ARTIFICIAL INSEMINATION

Q My husband is completely infertile, so it looks as though my only hope of having a baby is by artificial insemination. Do you think I could do this without telling him? And, if so, where could I get it done?

A To have artificial insemination by donor without telling your husband would be utter lunacy!

For a start, he presumably *knows* that he's completely infertile. He might just suspect something when

because it's almost unknown for the donor to be introduced to the couple. In most countries, the doctor will attempt to keep the man's identity a complete secret, though it has been suggested that proper registers of donors should be set up, so that the name of a donor could, if necessary, be checked at a later date.

Some doctors working in the field have allowed individual donors to father many children through insemination. But it's now increasingly felt that a young man who is a sperm donor should make only a few 'donations', *not* in order to save his strength for his medical studies, but to cut down on the risk of inter-marriage among the children he has sired.

There's now increasing emphasis on screening potential sperm donors to make sure that they're healthy (and don't have AIDS). But you have to bear in mind that in the unlikely event of the baby being born with some abnormality, there's no question of your having any legal redress, unless there has been some form of negligence.

As with AIH, the procedure for carrying out AID is very simple. The selected young man arrives at the clinic, and makes his 'donation' into a sterile container. It may be immediately frozen for use later. But it's possible that the doctor will have arranged for the donor to donate on the day that you're due to ovulate. You will come to the clinic a little later in the day, and the doctor will use a syringe to inject the sperm into the upper part of your vagina (the area of the cervix).

ARTIFICIAL INSEMINATION

you announce that you're in the family way. What he'll probably suspect is that you've been up to no good with the lodger!

No, if you're considering insemination then it can only be with your husband's agreement. A high proportion of infertile men *will* agree, if their wives talk it over with them carefully.

Q My husband has been told that he is completely sterile, so we have decided to have a baby by AID. Where can I get more information about this?

A You can get a leaflet about AID from BPAS – phone number 01-222 0985.

BO • BALDNESS • BEHAVIOUR THERAPY

Q I have a BO problem. People in the office have complained, and I feel that if I had a sexual relationship with a man, he would too! I've tried everything my doctors have suggested. Can you help?

A As a rather drastic solution, there is an operation to remove a saucer-sized area of skin from the armpits. This works very well – but it's painful!

Less drastic is a new invention for which great claims are being made. It's a battery-operated device which you place on the appropriate part of your body. The makers claim that it produces a temporary blockage of the sweat ducts, but you have to re-treat yourself every six weeks or so.

At present, it's unlikely to be available on the NHS, and it's pricey – £98 for the armpit model. More details from: John Bell and Croyden Ltd, *52–54 Wigmore Street, London W1H 0AU*. I wouldn't myself recommend buying such a device without clear proof that it works.

Q I read what you wrote about female baldness – pubic and otherwise. (See also PUBIC)

I'm a young woman and have suffered a lot of distress because of severe hair loss on my head. Is there any self-help group for sufferers?

A Yes: write (enclosing a large s.a.e.) to Hairline International, *Hill Vellacott, Post and Mail House, Colmore Circus, Birmingham, B4 6AT*. They're a support organisation for adults and children who've lost their hair.

I do hope that the new treatment called minoxidil (Regaine) will be able to help you get some of your hair back.

Q I am desperately shy. In fact I cannot even let my own husband see me without any clothes. My doctor said something called 'behaviour therapy' might help. Please can you explain more about this?

A Well, she's right. Behaviour therapy is a specific system of treatment which concentrates on helping you to find ways of altering

BLEEDING AFTER SEX • BREASTS

your symptoms — rather than digging around in your Freudian past! I've seen behaviourist seminars at which shy people are taught how to modify their own reactions — by role-plays, etc. And I'm sure the same thing could be done for your shyness about undressing. Your 'role-plays' for this could be quite something!

Q My husband's sperm has gone red. Is this OK?

A No, ma'am. This suggests that there's *bleeding* somewhere in his plumbing, and it must be investigated *soon*.

Your doctor will probably suggest that he goes to a urological surgeon for the necessary tests.

Q I have been a widow for five years, and have recently embarked on a love affair. After intercourse, I've been surprised to note a pink/red secretion. Is this just due to me being unaccustomed to lovemaking, or should I talk to my GP?

A This was almost certainly blood, and therefore you'd be best to have a check-up from a doctor. Indeed, *anyone* who bleeds post-coitally (especially after the menopause) would be wise to see her doctor.

But as you say, this may just have been due to the fact that you're a trifle out of practice. If so, a simple lubricant like KY or Durol (available at most chemists) would help until you've played yourself in.

Q I am 19 and since I lost my virginity a year ago, I have had (a) bleeding after every intercourse; (b) a yellow bubbly discharge, which has not got better on anti-thrush treatment from my doctor.

A The yellow, bubbly discharge is likely to be due to the infection called trichomonas. If your doc agrees, he/she will probably give you Flagyl tablets by mouth. Persistent bleeding after sex usually needs specialist investigation, but at your young age it is unlikely to be due to anything nasty.

Q I have recently heard of 'cystic breast disease'. As I have a hard lump in each breast, just

BREASTS

below the nipple, I feel I may have this. Do you think so?

A I beg you to see your doctor *urgently*. There's no way anyone can diagnose breast lumps except by examining them. Most likely these lumps are benign, but you *must* make sure.

This month I have several letters in my postbag from women who say they have breast lumps. The vital message which *every* woman should know is this: if you think you've noticed a lump in the breast, *always* have it checked out within a few days at most. Doing this could save your life.

Q I have what I think must be a fairly unusual complaint – my breasts are different sizes. I have met a man who I really care for, but I feel embarrassed at the thought of undressing in front of him. I have neither the means nor the inclination to submit to plastic surgery, so what can I do?

A This isn't all that unusual a problem. Many women have one breast which is much bigger than the other. But I do appreciate that this is deeply embarrassing for you. Really, the only cure would be by plastic surgery – which you might be able to get on the NHS.

If surgery's not your cup of tea, then you might be able to produce at least a slight improvement by regular and intensive exercise to build up the muscle behind the smaller breast.

The simplest way of doing this is just to put your hand on your hip bone, and press down very hard for about ten seconds. (This makes the muscle behind your breast stand out.) Relax for a few seconds – then repeat ten times.

As with any muscle-building exercise, you need to do it night and morning for about six months before you get any results. Very good luck to you.

Q My breasts are very small. Would hormone pills help?

A No – don't muck about with hormone pills, which could be dangerous. Really, the only way in which anyone can make any really significant increase in her boob size is through cosmetic surgery.

Q My teenage daughter has been horrified to discover that at the same time as her breasts developed, a third breast has appeared on the lower part of her

BREASTS

chest. There has always been a little brown mark on her skin there, but it now appears that this was a nipple.

We haven't told anybody else yet. Can anything be done?

APlease try and reassure your poor daughter that this condition is quite common, and can be very easily put right.

Having more than two breasts is called 'polymazia'. Famous sufferers have included Anne Boleyn, who is said to have had three. A woman whose case was recorded in a Victorian medical journal had nine, and another had an extra breast on her thigh!

But why does it happen? Look at a cat or a dog, and you'll see. They have a double row of teats, running down the chest and the abdomen. And just like them, human beings also have a streak of embryonic tissue which is called the 'milk line', which runs from the top of the chest down to the groin.

These extra nipples are perfectly harmless. But sometimes at

The Breast

The breast is a structure which, as you know, has always had enormous emotional importance for human beings. That breasts were regarded as supremely beautiful way back in Old Testament days is evidenced by the Song of Solomon: 'Thy two breasts are like two young roes that are twins, which feed among the lilies . . .'

To this day, men have tended to be obsessed with breasts; Freud (1856–1939) believed that boy babies learned their sexuality at their mothers' breasts, and that this explained the male fascination with the mammaries. (Where this leaves bottle-fed boy babies – and indeed girl babies – I don't know.)

Structure

Anyway, let's have a quick look at the basic anatomical structure of the human mammary.

The breast is a mass of milk gland tissue, embedded in fat, and set on the front of the muscular wall of the chest. From the glands which produce milk, a number of milk ducts (15 to 20) lead down to little milk sinuses (or collecting areas) just behind the nipple. In between the milk ducts, there's a network of fibrous tissue which gives the breast support – and also gives it that

162

BREAST CANCER

puberty one of them develops into a full-blown breast – which is what has happened with your daughter. Happily, this unwanted extra breast can be surgically removed. That's a job for a plastic surgeon, and your GP will be pleased to refer your daughter to one under the NHS.

Q I am 19, and have just found a lump in my right breast. Is this cancer?

firm, thrusting outline so beloved of adult males and babies. This fibrous tissue does tend to stretch with advancing years, particularly if the breasts are very big and heavy.

Size of the breasts depends on the amount of fat and glandular tissue contained in them, which is to a large extent controlled by the woman's own hormones. It's difficult and dangerous to achieve any change in breast size by giving hormone treatment. But nowadays it is not difficult to enlarge abnormally small breasts (or to reduce abnormally large ones) by plastic surgery.

A At your age, breast cancer is fantastically rare. (See page 24.) But any lump in the breast, at any age, should be examined by a doc.

Q As I've been on the Pill for four years, am I in danger of developing breast cancer?

A Research about the Pill and breast cancer is coming in very fast at the moment. Most of it is fairly reassuring, but there are disturbing suggestions that prolonged exposure to the Pill in younger women (especially those who have never been pregnant) may – and I repeat *may* be linked with breast cancer. But there are two factors which make it very difficult to assess th figures.

Firstly, the majority of cases of breast cancer occur in women aged 55-plus. At the moment, very few women over 55 have had much exposure to the Pill.

Secondly, in the case of most carcinogens (cancer-provoking agents), there's a 'time-lapse' of about 25 years after exposure, before the cancer occurs.

This means that because the Pill was scarcely used in Britain before about 1965, we wouldn't expect to see many Pill-induced cancers appearing till about now. ▶

BREAST CANCER

So I'm afraid we shall soon find out whether the Pill turns out to have been a boon to womankind – or the proverbial biological time-bomb.

AGE	CASES PER YEAR
15–19	1
20–24	15
25–29	107
30–34	376
35–39	750
40–44	1288
45–49	1744
50–54	1969
55–59	2411
60–64	2371
65–69 (PEAK)	2754
70–74	2575
75–79	2131
80–84	1472
85+	1200

Q I have just had a course of radiotherapy treatment following a 'lumpectomy' operation to remove a tumour from my breast. I am now feeling well and have been declared fit. But I am writing to make the point that when I first realised that I had a lump, I did not rush to the doctor (as I had always sworn that I would do in such circumstances). Indeed, when my doctor gave me a referral form to take to the hospital, I waited for a while before sending it off.

Disorders of the Breast

Cancer

What happens if you consult your doctor because you think you have found a lump? He will, of course, examine you himself to confirm that one is present. (Some women understandably mistake a slight thickening of the breast tissue for a lump.) Having assessed the swelling, he will arrange an urgent referral to a surgeon, who will usually perform a minor diagnostic operation on the breast within a few days.

This operation may just involve aspirating some fluid from the swelling with a needle – or it may involve taking away a tiny portion of the lump for examination under the microscope. These procedures will show if cancer is present. If it is, treatment will be started immediately.

The treatment of early breast cancer is nowadays fairly successful. This isn't the place to discuss the merits of the various methods of surgery and radiotherapy. Suffice it to say that the woman who has gone to her doctor *immediately* she has discovered a lump stands an

BREAST CANCER

excellent chance of living to a healthy old age.

Women tend, quite naturally, to be very frightened of the idea of losing a breast, but the courage that most women show in the face of this disease is quite remarkable.

N.B. Although breast cancer almost always makes its appearance in the form of a lump, it can sometimes cause other symptoms instead. The most common are *(i)* bleeding from the nipple, *(ii)* recent (as opposed to lifelong) inturning of the nipple, *(iii)* puckering of the skin of the breast, *(iv)* a raw, weepy area developing on the nipple.

Other Breast Conditions

SWELLINGS. There are many benign causes of lumps in the breast but, as explained above, tissue from all such lumps must be examined under the microscope within a matter of days. Removing a benign lump is a simple matter, and no further trouble need be anticipated after the operation.

OVER- AND UNDER-SIZED BREASTS. Many women are understandably dissatisfied with the size of their breasts. Where the bosom is very big or small, plastic surgery can sometimes help. Hormone creams should not be used, as they are dangerous. Many proprietary 'bust-developing' preparations are completely useless. The most popular 'bust-developer' in the world is, in fact, a simple exerciser, the object of which is to develop the muscles that lie behind the breast. It has at least the merit of being harmless!

MASTITIS. This means inflammation of the breasts. Most types of mastitis are fairly trivial, and respond moderately well to simple measures, such as wearing a better-fitting bra. Infective mastitis, however, will need antibiotic treatment and may progress to the stage of a breast abscess (*see* below).

BREAST ABSCESS. This is a common condition, at least during lactation. A painful swelling develops in the affected breast, and the overlying skin becomes reddened. Surgical opening of the abscess may be necessary, but in the early stages antibiotics alone may be sufficient.

BREAST CANCER

When my lump was eventually diagnosed as malignant the trauma was made worse by my feelings of anger with myself for not having acted with more urgency. I know that 'putting it off' is the most natural human reaction in such circumstances. But I am writing to urge you to continually remind your readers of the need for regular and constant self-examination, and the importance of getting treatment *immediately*, even if the doctor says (as mine did) 'It's probably nothing!'

A Quite right ma'am. There's nothing further to add to the point you have made so eloquently – so I'll just salute your courage, and thank you for taking the trouble to put this potentially life-saving advice on paper for the benefit of other readers.

Q I am 31, and very worried about cancer of the breast. I'd like to have a mammography screen, but my GP says the NHS can't afford it. Is this true?

A Regrettably, mammography (which is X-ray screening of the breast) isn't easily available in some areas of the country. But it is

Women: Care of Your Breasts, and Protecting Yourself Against Cancer

General care of the breasts isn't difficult: a straightforward wash with mild soap and water once a day is sufficient, followed by careful drying with a soft towel.

In late pregnancy and more especially early lactation, breasts and nipples need special care – mainly because cracks are liable to develop in the nipple. In the event of any cracking or soreness, apply a reliable antiseptic cream (your local pharmacist will advise you). If pain or even appreciable soreness develop, always consult your doctor or midwife.

Breast Cancer

It's a tragic and, to most people, unpalatable fact that breast cancer attacks roughly 1 out of every 17 women in western countries. (I can't help feeling that if cancer of the penis were as common in men, something would have been done about it by now!)

Many of these cases of breast

BREAST CANCER

cancer can be cured if caught early enough. X-ray screening for women is gradually being introduced. But at present it is only for the 50–64 age group. The fact is that for most women the best hope of catching the disease early is to detect it themselves.
Possible warning symptoms are:

- a *lump* (this may well not be cancerous, but should *always* be checked by a doctor)

- much less commonly, unexplained *bleeding* from the nipple

- occasionally, a *raw ulcer-like patch* of skin on the nipple

- sometimes, an unexplained *inturning of the nipple*

- unexplained *puckering of the skin* of the breast.

I should add that although many teenage girls and young women not unreasonably fear that they have breast cancer, it's primarily a disease of the over-30s – and is commonest in the over-50s. Cases occurring before the age of 25 do occur, but are very rare indeed.

The process of monthly self-examination for breast lumps is vitally important. (I'm not joking when I say that husbands and lovers can help here too, by looking out for lumps when they handle their loved ones' breasts.) An examination once a month should be sufficient. Feel all over the breast tissue, using the flat of the hands. If there is any lump present, **see your doctor within 24–48 hours.**

This breast check, should be a regular self-examination. The procedure is based on the splendid and underfunded work of the Women's National Cancer Control Campaign in Britain. An excellent leaflet describing the technique is available from WNCCC at *1 South Audley Street, London W1Y 5DQ* – enclose a large s.a.e. Follow it: it could save your life.

BREAST CANCER • BREAST IMPLANTS

supposed to be coming in for all women between 50 and 65.

If you feel you'd be happier having it done, then all I can suggest is that you ask your doc to refer you to one of the large private screening units run by organisations such as BUPA.

But let me make one important point. Few people have grasped that regular routine mammography only appears to be of value in women aged over about 45.

At the present moment, the best and most available defence against breast cancer for younger women seems to be to keep on examining your breasts for lumps once a month.

And of course, if you have the slightest suspicion of a lump – or anything else odd – in your breast, then I beg you to get a medical examination right away. Recent work suggests that many women are still waiting six or seven months before seeing a doctor – by which time it may be too late.

Q Although I like having my breasts handled, I am seriously concerned that this sort of manipulation could lead to breast cancer. Is this so?

A Fortunately, it's just a myth. Women who have their breasts handled a lot are *not* specially liable to breast carcinoma. For example, the incidence of this awful disease is far less in prostitutes than it is in nuns.

Q As a birthday present, my husband is going to pay for me to have plastic surgery to make my boobs bigger. Where could I get this done?

A Who's the birthday present for – you or him?

If you really want this done then good luck to you. However, it's important for you to realise that plastic surgery on the breast isn't always as successful as people think; so it's always best to go to a top-class, reputable plastic surgeon.

Where are you going to find one? Personally, I wouldn't recommend going off to one of the cosmetic surgery clinics which advertise in newspapers – unless you know that the clinic in question has a good local reputation. Nobody really controls the standards of these clinics, and some have been known to give people cross-eyed boobs!

Some clinics claim that they are 'approved by the Area Health Authorities' – which means virtually

BREAST IMPLANTS

nothing. Others announce that they only employ Fellows of the Royal College of Surgeons – which again doesn't mean much, because you don't need to have done any plastic surgery at all to become an FRCS.

So what's to be done? My own view is that in most instances it's best to begin by asking your own doc to refer you to a plastic surgeon. Though you'll obviously have to go privately, your GP might well choose a surgeon who is a consultant in plastic surgery at an NHS hospital. (Being a consultant at a large hospital is obviously a considerable guarantee of ability.)

Alternatively, there are now two organisations of surgeons who do this kind of work. If your doc doesn't know the address of a plastic surgeon, he or you can write to either of these organisations to obtain a list of names and addresses.

The two organisations are:

- The British Association of Aesthetic Plastic Surgeons, *c/o* The Royal College of Surgeons, Lincoln's Inn Fields, London WC2A 3PN.
- The British Association of Cosmetic Surgeons, *c/o* 7 Patterdale Road, Woodthorpe, Nottingham NG5 4LF.

Q I have always had one breast that is much, much smaller than the other, which has caused me terrible embarrassment. I have now been offered the chance of plastic surgery to implant a 'pad' into the smaller breast and make them the same size. Should I go ahead?

A Yes. All surgery carries a slight risk. But if you really feel bad about the fact that you're a bit like the young lady of Devizes (whose boobs were of differing sizes), then go ahead and have the op.

Q For all my adult life I have been deeply unhappy about my almost completely flat chest. (Currently, I have difficulty filling a 30AA bra.) Small fortunes spent on creams and potions and hours of 'bust-building' exercises have been to no avail. For many years now I have thought about having a boob job done, but the high cost made this an impossibility. However, I am finally in a financial position to afford it. How can I go about finding a good cosmetic surgeon? Please don't tell me to forget all about it, or start expounding the everybody's beautiful in their own way theory!

BREAST IMPLANTS

A I wouldn't dream of it: flat boobs can make a woman feel as though nature's dealt her a lousy hand. However, I'm not too happy about some of these cosmetic surgery clinics which advertise to the public; you may end up getting your breasts operated on by a dentist (seriously), so write to the addresses on the previous page.

Q A few years ago I had breast implants to increase my bust size. It was one of the best things I've ever done, and has given me great self-confidence.

But this year I'm going on holiday abroad, and will be flying for the first time. Is it true that people who have had breast implants should not fly, because the implants can explode at altitude?

A In the early days of breast enlargement, there were one or two reports of implants going 'pop' when the airliner reached about 40,000 feet. But this just doesn't seem to happen today – perhaps because surgeons use a better class of implant.

However, I should point out to you that 'falsies' (inflatable brassières filled with air) can and do explode in the low-pressure atmosphere of an aircraft. Travellers who rely on pneumatic devices to boost their bustlines should discreetly let out a little air in the Departure Lounge.

THE CAP

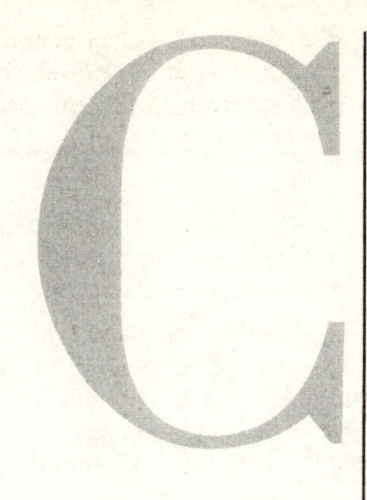

Q I am getting fed up with the Pill, which makes me feel depressed and bloated.
Is the cap any good?

A Yes, jolly good method, the cap. If you use it properly, it's nearly as effective as the Pill.

Also, it has practically no side effects — except that urinary infections (like cystitis) seem to be more common in cap-users.

All Family Planning clinics fit caps, so get yourself down there and get measured up for one of the correct size.

Q You will probably think me very haughty, but I do have several lovers, who do not know about one another. For contraception, I rely on the cap. Would it be better if I used a different one for each lover?

A Goodness, you do seem to be living life in the fast lane. Anyway, the cap (diaphragm) is designed to fit the woman — not the man. So there is no need to have a separate one for each gent.

Perhaps you were worried about the hygiene of using the same diaphragm for each man? As a

THE CAP • CANCER OF THE CERVIX

rule, most women take out their caps about eight hours after intercourse, then wash and dry them. This procedure will give perfectly adequate hygiene, provided you can fit it into your schedule.

The Cap (Diaphragm)

The cap or diaphragm has become more popular in recent years, probably as a result of various pill scares. The most widely used contraceptive cap is a simple disc of rubber. The idea is that a woman slips it into her vagina *so that it covers her* cervix (the neck of her womb). Before putting it in, she coats it with a contraceptive cream or gel.

Rather surprisingly *neither she nor her partner should be able to feel the device once it's in position.* So a well-fitted cap shouldn't interfere with lovemaking in any way.

The important words here are 'well-fitted'. Women's vaginas vary substantially in size, so you must be fitted (by a doctor) with the size of cap which is right for you. Equally importantly, you have to be taught how to put the device in correctly before lovemaking, and how to take it out the following morning.

The cap *must* be inserted so that it covers the cervix – otherwise it will be quite useless.

When the cap fails to protect against pregnancy, the usual reason is that the woman has been putting it in the wrong place – usually in *front* of her cervix. So it's very important to be sure that you understand your own anatomy before you rely on this method.

Note: there are some rarer types of cap available in Britain and other countries (not widely in the USA) for women whose vaginal muscles are too lax for an ordinary diaphragm. Several new types of cap have also been invented recently.

Q I had six or seven lovers when I was younger, including a couple of 'one-night stands'. I presume from what I have read that this means I am likely to get cancer of the cervix. Am I right?

CANCER OF THE CERVIX

A No, ma'am — you're not. I keep trying to make clear in this column that cancer of the cervix *isn't* just 'caused by sex', as you might think from reading some newspapers.

It appears to be linked with a number of factors, which include the pill, smoking, social class, geographical location, race — and whether your partner (or possibly yourself) is involved in manual labour.

In other words, it's still a mystery! But certainly, your chances of developing it are increased if: (a) You've had multiple sex partners; or (b) Your husband has had multiple sex partners.

In your particular case, the fact that you've had what us doctors euphemistically describe these days as 'a number of boyfriends' *doesn't* mean that you're certain to get cervical cancer — though, like everyone else, you should have regular smears.

One final point: the current publicity over cancer of the cervix has led many people to think, like yourself, that the chances of dying from it are high.

This isn't so. One woman in 150 dies from cervical cancer. One woman in every 30 dies from lung cancer — and one in every 23 from breast cancer.

The last two are REALLY common causes of cancer deaths in women, and it's a great pity that more isn't being done to prevent them. (If I were prime minister, I'd start off by jailing a few tobacco manufacturers!)

Q My ex-wife has developed cancer of the cervix.

I'm very worried about the theory that this is caused by a germ. Could I have transmitted it to other women I've made love to? And should I contact them to warn them?

A That's very thoughtful of you. The 'germ theory' of cancer of the cervix is still unproven. Also, if you have been a reasonably hygienic chap (in other words, if you wash your penis each day) that lessens the chance of having passed anything on.

But I think it'd be reasonable if you indicated to your lovers — without alarming them — that they should have regular smear tests. If they do that it's very unlikely that they'll be in danger.

Q I am in my mid-30s and have just had a routine smear which revealed I have 'mild dysplasia'.

The doctor told me that this is the

173

CANCER OF THE CERVIX

pre-cancerous phase. I am feeling very unhappy, and wondering how my husband and small children will manage without me when I am gone.

How can I have got this cancer, as I thought it related to promiscuity? I have never slept with anyone apart from my husband.

A First thing to say, ma'am, is that there has been some massive misunderstanding here. You have nothing to worry about, and are not going to die.

'Mild dysplasia' is a common finding, which means that the cells could well become cancerous if left long enough. They may get better over the next few years — but if they don't, a simple operation will cure you. So cheer up!

Second thing to say is that a lot of people seem to have got this idea that you can't get cancer or pre-cancer unless you've slept around. That's a load of old-rhubarb (as we doctors say).

There are other factors, such as smoking, having had several babies, and being married to someone in a manual job.

Q I work in a hospital cytology department, and I noted with interest your comments on cervical screening in SHE (in which you complained about the lack of availability of smear tests for British women).

Surely the majority of women who die from cervical cancer have not had the test because they did not come forward for it — and not because the test was unavailable to them?

A I must admit, sir, that there's some truth in what you say: many women have the opportunity of having the smear test, but either refuse it or else don't bother.

On the other hand, there are plenty of women who have great difficulty in getting a smear done. And there are a lot of others (particularly in the poorer areas of Britain) who've never had a smear because our creaking NHS has never offered them one.

Q Would my doctor remember to let me know if my smear test showed cancer? I have always had regular smears, and thought I was safe. But I have been horrified to read that women may have died because doctors didn't tell them their test results.

A Well, I've been saying for years in SHE that our national smear test system is a muddle and

CANCER OF THE CERVIX

The Cervix

Every woman should be familiar with her own cervix – after all, if a man can touch your cervix, why shouldn't you?

But, what *is* the cervix?

As you probably know, it's widely referred to as 'the neck of the womb'. But really it's the *tip* of the womb, the very point of the womb, which projects down a few centimetres into the vagina.

A narrow tunnel runs up through the cervix and into the cavity of the womb itself. This is the only way into the womb from the exterior. Sperms pass up through this canal into the womb immediately after intercourse. Naturally, menstrual blood passes down through it at period times.

And, of course, during childbirth the baby has to pass through this hole through the middle of the cervix. Fortunately, the cervix has the remarkable property of opening up to a quite extraordinary extent during labour – so that the previously-narrow tunnel becomes wide enough to let the baby's head go through it. (It shrinks' down almost to the same size as before, very soon after childbirth.)

Functions

It's difficult to say what the *function* of the cervix is – except to provide a useful sort of expandable entrance and exit to the womb.

Some women do derive considerable sexual pleasure from having it touched – particularly during the last 'surge' of intercourse – but others don't have any special feeling there.

This may be owing to individual variations in nerve supply to the cervix. Certainly, it's a remarkable fact that while many women feel *pain* when a surgical instrument has to be applied to the cervix, a whopping minority of the female population feel absolutely no painful sensation at all.

In this century, the cervix has developed one important new function – as a sort of useful hat-peg on which to hang a contraceptive cap. Any woman with a cap *must* be able to feel her cervix with her fingertips.

CANCER OF THE CERVIX

a disgrace – and now I'm afraid that the chickens are beginning to come home to roost.

Among the general shambles, a small number of women have not been told that their tests were positive. The odds against this happening are very long. But when it *does* happen, a woman may lose her life unnecessarily.

In the present confusion, my advice to all adult women is this. It's wildly unlikely that your doctor would fail to tell you that your smear test was positive. But just in case, you can protect yourself by asking for the result at your doctor's surgery or clinic, about six to eight weeks after having the test.

Disorders of the Cervix

CANCER OF THE CERVIX

Any woman (especially one who has not recently had a satisfactory smear) should watch out for the following symptoms:

Bleeding after intercourse

Bleeding between periods

Unexplained pain in the pelvic region, including pain on intercourse.

See your doctor within a few days, even if bleeding is confined to a few spots of blood or a faint brownish discharge. He should do an internal examination, look at the cervix and probably refer you to a gynaecologist – unless there's some obvious reason, such as that the contraceptive Pill you're taking doesn't suit you.

CERVICITIS. A form of inflammation which is quite common. The principal symptom is discharge. Simple local treatment as an outpatient is usually curative.

CERVICAL EROSION. This is a trivial complaint which can produce slight vaginal bleeding and discharge. It often occurs after childbirth. Treatment is hardly ever necessary unless an erosion produces pain on intercourse or a trying amount of discharge. In these cases, 'cautery' (with a chemical or hot or cold probe) should give a rapid and virtually painless cure.

POLYPS OF THE CERVIX. These occur at all ages, and cause discharge and slight bleeding. Removal is very easy.

CANCER OF THE CERVIX

Q I am worried about the possibility of getting cancer of the cervix. How can I find out when my next smear test is due?

A A simple way of finding out when your next smear is due is this:

In most parts of this country, your test will be recorded on a rectangular form, about the size of this page. The lab usually puts in the suggested date for your next smear on the form.

One copy of the form is sent to your GP, and one to whoever did the test (if it was done by someone other than your doctor).

At present, I'm afraid that the form is tending to take something like six to eight weeks to be returned to your doctor or clinic. So what you need to do is to contact your GP or clinic at the end of that time — and ask to be told the suggested date which has been written in on the form.

Q After reading many books and articles on the subject of cervical cancer, I find there's one question which still troubles me. As there now appears to be a great deal of evidence to show that the precursors of cancer of the cervix may be transmitted from the penis to the vagina, is there a danger of contracting carcinomas of the mouth or throat through oral sex?

A At the moment, there's no known relationship between oral love play and cancer of the mouth or throat. In fact oral or throat cancers are often closely linked with smoking — especially pipe-smoking — or with ill-fitting dentures rubbing on a sore place for many years.

Alcohol may play a part, and the oriental habit of chewing betel-nut is also said to be a factor in some cases. But often the cause isn't known. Mouth cancers actually seem to have become rarer during the course of this century, and standard surgical textbooks attribute this to the decline in clay pipe smoking.

In spite of the fact that there's now so much oral love play around, there's no suggestion that oral cancers are on the increase. But as with other forms of sex, it's very important to cut down all possible risks by being hygienic. No woman should do fellatio for a feller unless she's sure that he's clean and washed!

Q I am terrified about the prospect of getting cancer of the cervix. Is it true that there's some

CANCER OF THE CERVIX

birth control method that would protect me?

A Yes – both the sheath and the diaphragm (cap) are thought to give a woman some degree of protection against cervical cancer.

Q My husband and I are in our mid-50s, and have a wonderful sex life, including oral sex. But he is a heavy smoker, and I'm worried that this could give me cervical cancer.

A I don't think your husband's smoking is likely to give you cervical cancer. The only known connection between the disease and smoking is that it is more common in smokers.

This may just be owing to two factors:

Cancer of the cervix is much commoner down in socio-economic groups IV and V (a fact which isn't widely publicised, because people are embarrassed about talking about 'class' these days).

Smoking is *also* more common in this section of the population.

There is no proof that smoking *causes* cancer of the cervix. Unfortunately, there is now no doubt whatever that smoking causes cancer of the lung (which kills 16 times as many people as cancer of the

Protecting Yourself Against Cervical Cancer

In most western countries, cervical cancer kills nearly as many women as road accidents do. But in many poorer countries, the death rate is much higher.

I cannot emphasise too strongly that:

all women (except virgins) are at risk

the disease is *preventable*.

We still don't really know why cancer of the cervix occurs. It certainly has a link with sex – and this is the aspect that the newspapers usually stress!

It's true that it only occurs in women who have had sex – and that it seems to be a bit more common in women who have had several lovers.

On the other hand, the newspapers rarely mention that this appalling killer is also more common in:

smokers

CANCER OF THE CERVIX

cervix), so I must be blunt and say that it's your husband – not you – who is in danger.

less well-off women

women who've had children

women over 35

women living in certain geographical areas.

But as I've said, *all* women who've ever had sex (even if it's only with their husbands) are liable to it. So unless you've led a totally celibate life (in which case, you're unlikely to be reading this book), *you owe it to yourself to take precautions against it.*

What precautions? Well first of all there's now considerable evidence that *barrier* methods of contraception (the cap or diaphragm, and the sheath) help protect a woman against cancer of the cervix.

Secondly, almost all doctors now agree that *all* adult women who have ever had sex should make sure they have regular smear tests.

In a smear test, all that happens is that the doctor uses a wooden spatula to scrape some cells off the cervix (the neck of the womb). The doctor puts these on a glass slide, and sends it to the laboratory for microscopic examination.

The point of the whole thing is this: *if there are any abnormal cells present, this gives very, very early warning of the disease – long before it causes any symptoms.* And at that stage, it's nearly always curable by laser therapy or a small biopsy ('sampling') operation.

Cancer of the cervix does eventually produce symptoms, but by the time it produces these symptoms, it's awfully late in the day. It's far, far better to detect it 10 or 20 years beforehand by the simple and – in most cases – painless technique of a smear test.

CANCER OF THE CERVIX • CHLAMYDIA

Q I'm very worried about the possibility of getting cancer of the cervix, because I have just realised that I am in one of the 'at risk' groups. This is because I had sex with a boy when I was a young teenager.

I am now 24, and the only other man I have slept with has been my husband.

A Then relax, ma'am. I keep trying to point out in this column that there are plenty of other 'risk factors' apart from having had teenage sex, for instance having dozens of lovers, being a manual worker, being a smoker.

And though cancer of the cervix can be awful if it's not 'caught' early, only one woman in 125 dies from this cause. The death figures for other tumours (such as cancer of the breasts or lungs) are far higher.

Also, I'd like to point out that at 24 time is very much on your side. Although the newspapers keep rabbiting on about 'epidemics' of cervical cancer in young women, you may be surprised to learn that the peak age for this disease is between 55 and 59!

I admit that there has been a worrying increase in cases in younger women lately. But if you have regular smear tests, the chance of you coming to any harm as a result of your teenage love affair is very, very small indeed.

Chlamydia

This is a 'new' infection, in the sense that it wasn't discovered all that long ago, and many people have never heard of it.

Yet millions of women worldwide have it – and in many cases it has affected their tubes and made them infertile. Regrettably, inexpensive tests for chlamydia aren't yet widely available (it doesn't show up on ordinary swabs). The result is that the condition often goes undiagnosed.

Chlamydia should be suspected if a woman has persistent vaginal/pelvic pain, with or without a fever and a discharge. Salpingitis (see below) may be present. It's vitally important to get treatment with the right antibiotic – penicillin is useless, but erythromycin or tetracycline usually work.

CIRCUMCISION • THE CLITORIS

Circumcision

Circumcision remains popular in America, and in Jewish and Moslem cultures — but it's not very popular elsewhere. In Britain, less than 7% of all male babies are now circumcised — partly because of worries about the horrendous damage which can be done by a badly-performed circumcision (e.g. partial amputation of the penis).

However, circumcision does make it easier to keep the male organ clean, and so greatly cuts down on the risk of cancer of the penis in later life.

Most adults will have had the decision about circumcision taken for them by their parents. So the only point I want to make here is this: Dr Kinsey discovered that in many adult males, the foreskin will not 'go back' (or 'unpeel') when the penis is erect. That isn't a good state of affairs — either sexually or hygienically!

So if *your* foreskin is too tight to go back properly, then you owe it to yourself and your partner to see a doctor and have a circumcision done. Provided you consult an experienced surgeon, you should find this a relatively painless operation.

Q I feel abnormal, a freak, and a total failure as a woman. This is because of the fact I was born with a clitoris which is positioned outside my vagina. I've always felt that no man would ever find me attractive in bed because of this, so I've always turned them down.

Now I've fallen in love with the nicest man I've ever met. Yet I can't face the possibility of him rejecting me if he saw me naked.

Could I have an operation to make me normal? This is the most difficult letter I've ever written.

A Well, thank heavens you wrote! For I've got good news for you: the clitoris is *supposed* to be outside the vagina. It's tragic that you've spent so many years of unhappiness because of this misunderstanding about basic female anatomy.

A woman's clitoris is actually located well above the opening of her vagina, just in front of her pubic bone.

You desperately need some reassurance about your own anatomy. In your letter you say that you

THE CLITORIS • COLPOSCOPY

don't want to go to your own doc – so I suggest you get yourself examined by a woman medical officer at a family planning clinic. I'm sure she'll be very willing to check out your clitoris (and surrounding bits), and confirm that they're quite OK. Good luck.

Q I recently had a smear which was not quite right, so I went to a gynaecologist who did something called a 'colposcopy'.

He said everything was OK now, but can I trust him?

The Clitoris

From studying overseas editions of previous books of mine, I have been able to discover what the clitoris is called in various tongues. In German, it's *die Kitzler*, in Dutch it's *de clitoris*, in French it's *le cli-cli* – and in the Hebrew edition of one of my books it's represented by something that looks like the figures '72727', followed by a picture of Stonehenge!

The clitoris is located just in front of the pubic bone – so it will be gently compressed and squeezed during intercourse. It's only the size of a little button – even when it swells up during sexual excitement. Close examination of it reveals that it's in fact very similar in structure to a man's penis, so it's not surprising that it's more plentifully supplied with 'pleasure-producing' nerve endings than any other part of the female body.

Male readers may like to note that during love-play, many women (not all) do prefer to be stimulated along the *side* of the clitoris, rather than directly on top of it.

Disorders

Disorders of the clitoris are very rare. Occasionally, women seek medical advice because of a sudden and alarming *swelling* of the clitoris. This swelling appears to be due to a collection of blood – and it soon bursts, leaving no ill-effects.

Some years ago, I described the condition in *World Medicine*, and promptly received a number of letters from doctors who had also seen it. Two of them had discovered that their patients had actually caused the swelling by wrapping a cotton thread round the clitoris during masturbation – clearly, this is *not* a very sensible idea!

CONCEPTION

A Yup. A colposcopy is just like having your cervix examined by a very powerful pair of opera glasses. The great magnification gives the specialist an excellent idea of what's happening in the area where cancer is liable to develop.

The fact that you were able to get a colposcopy at all is *good* – many areas don't have this equipment. Be reassured; but keep on having smears at the intervals recommended by the doc.

Q I'm 45, and suddenly want to have a child for the first time. Is conception possible at this age? And if so, what are the possible risks which could affect the child?

A Yes, conception is usually possible in your 40s – though your fertility may well be much less than it was when you were in your 20s.

The main risk to the baby is that of Down's syndrome, which occurs with roughly this frequency:

Women under 30	1 in 1200
Women 40+	1 in 100
Women 45+	1 in 50

I hope you succeed in having a baby. Have fun trying.

Q Is it true that I will have more chance of having a baby if my husband dips his balls in very cold water immediately before we start to make love?

We have been trying for nearly a year, but have had absolutely no luck, so are willing to give anything a go.

A Well, as a general rule, men do produce more sperm if their testicles are cool.

That's why blokes with a low sperm count are usually advised to avoid getting over-heated – for instance, to steer clear of hot, nylon jockey-shorts, which raise the scrotal temperature to quite alarming heights!

It's true that some people have gone so far as to advise would-be fathers to increase their chances of conception by cooling down their wotsits.

The late, great Kenneth More popularised this technique on TV by talking about it when he and his wife were trying for a child.

But I'm afraid that dipping the testicles in icy water *just before making love* would be pointless (as well as being decidedly uncomfortable – for both of you!).

You see, sperm take many weeks to develop inside the testes. So 'ball-freezing' would have no

CONCEPTION

effect on the sperm-count until about six weeks later.

If your man wants to dash out and sit in the December snow, that *might* improve his sperm count round about January or February. But it would be more sensible to go to an Infertility Clinic a.s.a.p. and try to find out *why* the pair of you have been having trouble conceiving.

Q Could the TB which I had many years ago be responsible for my current failure to conceive?

A Yes, possibly – TB can block the tubes. If you don't conceive fairly soon, seek help at an infertility clinic.

Q I am 24 years of age, married, and would love a baby – but after having tried for one for almost a year now, I am becoming rather worried. What should I do?

A If you've been trying for a year, then I think it's time to get some expert help.

Your GP may well be willing to do some initial tests (which I'll explain in a moment). If not, then try your local family planning clinic. If the initial tests don't reveal a cause for the difficulty in conceiving, then you and your husband will need to go to an infertility clinic for more sophisticated investigations. Initial tests include:

An internal examination of the woman

A brief physical check-up on the man

A sperm count on the man

A daily temperature chart kept by the woman for about six months – to try to see if she's ovulating

Possibly a post-coital test – in which the woman is examined internally soon after making love (to see how the sperms are getting on inside her)

Whichever doctor you see should also make some sort of inquiry to ensure that you're both 'doing it right'. Many couples aren't.

For instance, I recently came across a case in which a woman had undergone thousands of pounds' worth of time-consuming and uncomfortable investigations, which had shown she was perfectly normal. She had been too embarrassed to tell the specialist the real cause of the trouble – which was the fact that her husband couldn't get a good enough erection to get inside her.

CONCEPTION • CONTRACEPTION

Q I've just acquired an older lover. He says he needn't use a condom, as he couldn't possibly get anybody pregnant at his age.

But what is the oldest age at which a man has fathered a baby?

A 104. So unless your lover is at least 105 years old, he'd better 'don the con'!

Q Could I possibly get pregnant if my husband 'comes' outside me?

What worries me is that I might conceive if some sperm on a sheet got into my vagina.

A Just about possible, ma'am. A few cases of so-called 'virgin births' occur because the man's sperm gets deposited on a sheet or a thigh – and is transferred accidentally to the vagina (most often on the fingertips).

But once semen has dried out on a sheet, it's practically impossible for it to fertilise you.

Q I'm 35, and have an elderly 'boyfriend' of 71. Would a man of over 70 be able to father a child?

A Most definitely. Plenty of *over-80s* have done it – including Charlie Chaplin!

And in Elizabethan days, an old bloke called Thomas Parr got a poor serving wench with child at the age of 104 (him, not her).

Anyway, that was what she claimed – and he was probably too proud of himself to dispute it!

Q Is it possible for a woman to get pregnant if the man does not penetrate her, but simply comes outside?

A Yup. This is the explanation of a number of cases of alleged 'virgin birth' which have turned up in the Sunday newspapers over the years. (Some of them have been virgin on the ridiculous.)

Q Would the new contraceptive pill, called 'Dianette', help my spots and acne?

A Probably – but discuss it carefully with your doc first, as it's fairly powerful.

CONDOM • CONTRACEPTION

Condom

Although a lot of people are put off by the idea of the sheath, there is no doubt that it's one of the most popular and effective methods of contraception in the world. In most western countries, it's only just behind the Pill in the popularity stakes – and if there are any more Pill scares, it will probably regain the Number One position that it had in pre-Pill days.

I believe that more women should insist on their partners wearing a sheath – especially as, unlike the Pill or the IUD, it has virtually no side-effects. (A very few people are allergic to rubber, or to chemicals used in the process of vulcanization of rubber – but they can use 'hypo-allergenic' sheaths.)

There's also the very important plus-point that a sheath (like a diaphragm) probably helps to protect a woman against cancer of the cervix. It also gives at least some protection against any possible infection.

Indeed, sheaths are so useful that a small but increasing number of independent-minded women do carry them themselves for their own protection – and if they decide to go to bed with a lover, they make sure he uses one!

Some men who are having a bit of trouble with their potency do find it a little difficult to put a condom on – indeed, it's really quite common for women to say to a doctor, 'We can't use the sheath, because my husband can't get on with it . . .'

The answer to this problem is to make the putting on of the sheath *a part of love-play*. In other words, the woman can stimulate the man's penis with her hands until it's really hard. Then she can gently unroll the condom onto it. *That* usually solves the problem.

Note that sheath manufacturers have at last cottoned on to the

Q Is it true that there's some new French tablet that brings on your period each month, so you don't have to worry about using contraception?

A Yes, there is a French tablet called RU468, which does something rather like what you say. I have occasionally conversed on the phone – in broken French –

CONTRACEPTION

idea of making sheaths that will give women pleasure. They now make condoms with gentle 'ribbing' on the sides, so as to increase vaginal stimulation. Some women also appreciate the new coloured condoms, which look a lot better than the rather unattractive khaki shades of yesteryear.

Finally, it has to be admitted that sheaths do sometimes break. For that reason, many family planning specialists do recommend that you use a spermicide as an added precaution.

Some sheaths are now supplied with a pre-added spermicide. Alternatively, you can buy and use a *separate* spermicidal preparation. In Britain, it is common for a couple to insert a spermicidal pessary (vaginal tablet) about 10 minutes before intercourse: in America and some other countries, a spermicidal aerosol foam is more common.

with its inventor, Professor Etienne Baulieu, and he prefers to regard RU468 as 'an effective and safe method for termination of very early pregnancy' which can be used at the time the period is first noticed to be overdue.

But RU468 tends to cause heavy and prolonged bleeding, so it's not yet licensed for general use in Britain. If it is released in this country, there is bound to be a storm of moral outrage, because it could give every woman the power to abort herself each month if she wants to.

Q My wife and I have a very 'open' marriage, but of course I wouldn't like her to become pregnant by any of the other men she makes love with.

Our problem may strike you as silly, but we are too embarrassed to ask our doctor about it. Is it all right for her to use the same contraceptive 'cap' for each man? Or should she have a separate one for each person she sleeps with?

A There is no need for your wife to keep a separate cap for each bloke. Her life sounds quite complicated enough as it is, without having the additional problem of trying to remember which diaphragm she's supposed to be using.

But I think you and your wife should bear in mind that the cap does have a small failure rate – usually reckoned as about four

CONTRACEPTION

pregnancies per 100 women per year.

If she does fall pregnant, you're certainly going to have a heck of a time working out who the father is.

Q I would really like to try that new contraceptive sponge you mentioned a long time ago in SHE. Is there any news of it being available in Britain yet?

A A lot of women are interested in the new vaginal sponge — probably for aesthetic reasons, because it isn't messy, and is a nice, 'feminine' thing to use.

It is now available over the counter in Britain, under the brand name 'Today'.

But here's the bad news. Attractive as this new method of contraception seems to be, the results of British trials have not been encouraging. In one test, no less than 25 out of 126 women became pregnant while using the sponge!

So I think that you should consider very carefully before deciding to rely completely on this new method for your protection.

Q I have recently had a mastectomy, because of breast cancer. This is enough to cope with on its own, but I find my main problem is with contraception. Having been advised to keep off the Pill

Cystitis

This means inflammation of the bladder, but in some cases which are labelled 'cystitis' there is inflammation of the rest of the urinary passages and even of the kidneys too. For this reason, cystitis is not entirely the trivial 'chill' that many people imagine it to be. In recent years, it has become clear that cystitis, unless properly treated, can sometimes have serious consequences on the kidneys.

The symptoms of cystitis are *pain on passing water* and *a frequent desire to do so*. There is sometimes a little blood in the urine. Quite often, these symptoms follow a woman's first experiences of love-making ('honeymoon cystitis').

As a general rule, cystitis is due to infection by germs which have entered the opening of the urinary passage (the urethra) and made their way up to the bladder.

In women, this passage is very, very short and, of course, very near the rectum — from which most such germs come. This is

CONTRACEPTION • CYSTITIS

(because I have had breast cancer) I went to a Family Planning Clinic to have a cap fitted.

However, as I am overweight, the doctor there said she couldn't fit either the cap or the coil because of the difficulty in finding my cervix!

So, am I to become resigned to

---

why cystitis is very common in women but very rare in men (except those with prostate trouble) – in fact, a man who developed cystitis without apparent reason would need a careful investigation of his urinary system, including X-rays, to see if some structural abnormality was present.

Treatment, if it's to be effective, has to be vigorous! It's certainly not sufficient to go along and ask the doctor for a bottle of medicine, and then forget about the whole thing if the symptoms go off in a couple of days.

Nowadays, the doctor will usually send a specially collected specimen of urine to the lab before he starts treatment – often a 10-day course of antibiotics. The result of this test will (with luck) let him know whether he's got you on the right antibiotic.

Incidentally, until the antibiotic starts working, you can relieve your pain by drinking plenty of liquid, putting a hot-water bottle over your bladder, and taking a little bicarbonate of soda.

However, the world-famous 'Kilmartin self-help regime' says that you should also:

avoid bubble baths and all other possible chemical irritants

wash your genital area daily with a clean cloth which you boil after use – and keep for no other purpose

in the event of an attack of cystitis, take a painkiller

then drink plenty of water with a level teaspoon of bicarbonate of soda

finally, apply one hot-water bottle to your lower abdomen, and place another one between your thighs.

Remember too that as cystitis is so very often started off by love-play or love-making (and especially by *inept* efforts at love-play), it's a good idea to insist that your partner is gentle, careful and clean when he handles this delicate area of your body.

CONTRACEPTION • CYSTITIS

using sheaths? This must be a common problem for 'mastectomees', since we are told that we should not become pregnant for five years after having breast cancer.

Yes, this is indeed a common problem, ma'am — and thank you for your very jolly and cheerful letter, which must have been written in the face of some adversity (to put it mildly).

Roughly one woman in every 15 develops breast cancer, and most of those who have the misfortune to get it do have some form of mastectomy operation.

Since breast cancer is usually a 'hormone-dependent' growth, it's true that (as you say) most patients are advised not to use the Pill afterwards. For the same reasons, most women are advised by their surgeons not to become pregnant for some years after having the cancer removed.

So what are all these thousands of women going to use for birth control after the operation? For it's important to realise that most of them are, like yourself, interested in sex — and sexually attractive — despite having been ill.

The basic choices left are:

1 the sheath;
2 the coil (IUD);
3 the cap (diaphragm);
4 the new chemical sponge (which will be available by the time this appears in print);
5 vasectomy;
6 female sterilisation;
7 some variation of the rhythm method ('safe period').

I *haven't* included either the mini-Pill (progestogen-only Pill) or 'the shot' (the contraceptive injection), because there are considerable doubts as to whether they should be given to women who've had breast cancer.

If you don't want to have any more children, then you and your husband should seriously consider vasectomy or female sterilisation. But if you *do* want more babies, the choice lies between methods 1, 2, 3, 4 and 7. With all due respect to the doctor who has examined you, I don't think that method 2 (the coil) and method 3 (the cap) are necessarily ruled out because of the difficulty in finding your cervix.

Certainly, you can't use a cap till somebody has taught you to find your own cervix. But a doctor who is very experienced in IUD work ought to be able to find your cervix and insert a coil for you. Ask your own GP for the name of someone in your area who is practised in difficult IUD insertions.

Good luck.

CYSTITIS

Q From the moment I first had sex, I have been plagued with cystitis. Each act of intercourse makes it worse, and my GP seems to be unable to do anything about it.

A Discuss with him or her whether the time has now come for a referral to a urologist.

Q I see that you have had a lot of letters from cystitis sufferers. I don't know whether you think this would help, but I found that both myself and my daughter were cured of cystitis when we stopped eating pears. Do you think that cystitis could be due to an allergy to pears?

A I don't know – but certainly food sensitivities now seem to be much more common than was previously thought. So cystitis sufferers might like to try avoiding pears, and see what happens. Incidentally, some women with cystitis seem to do better if they avoid alcohol.

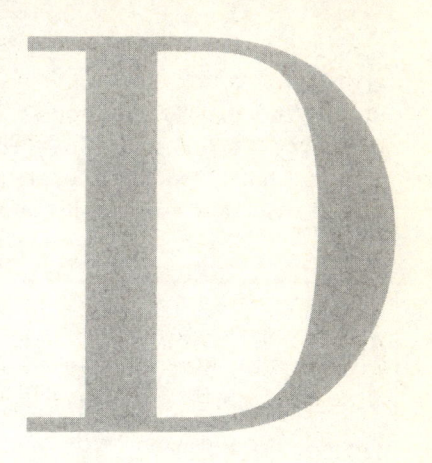

DIET • D & C

Q What exactly is a 'D and C'? My doctor said I needed one, and has given me a letter to take to a surgeon to have it done. But when I asked him what it was, he just laughed and said it was 'a sort of de-coke of the engine'.

A Um, yes – us male docs do

Diet

Yes – diet and your sex life are linked! If you let your body become obese and out of shape, you'll probably damage your sex life.

Also, good nutrition does seem to have a beneficial effect on most human activities – and it seems highly probable that it's good for sexual activity too. At present, the best medical opinion is that if you want a good all-round diet, you should eat plenty of the following:

green vegetables (including peas, beans, lettuce, cabbage, cauliflower and spinach)

root vegetables (carrots, turnips, swede and potatoes – yes, potatoes!)

fish

wholemeal bread

fruit

Despite what manufacturers say, you should try and steer clear of too much:

salt

butter

cheese

fried food

fatty meats

cream

anything that contains saturated (mainly animal) fats – including pastry and cookies

alcohol – especially spirits.

It's a bit hard to say whether *sugar* should be added to this list. Certainly, sugar is nowhere near as fattening as most people imagine – but it does provide 'empty' calories (which seem to be of no real nutritional value).

Also – despite the understandable efforts of the sugar industry to convince us otherwise – it

D & C

tend to make unfortunate remarks like that. Anyway, let me try to explain it a bit more fully. A D and C is the commonest operation performed in this country, with about 140,000 women undergoing the procedure each year. The initials stand for 'dilatation and curettage' – and what *that* means is: widening the channel through the neck of the womb so that an instrument can be passed through it; using the aforesaid instrument to curette – scrape out – the lining of the womb. A D and C is very often known simply as 'a scrape'.

It can be useful as a means of diagnosing womb disorders, because it enables surgeons to take out pieces of womb lining and examine them under the microscope.

Also, it can be an effective form of treatment (as opposed to diagnosis) for some womb conditions. For example, a D and C is an efficient way of removing pieces of afterbirth (placenta), which are often left behind after childbirth or miscarriage.

In Britain, the procedure is almost invariably done under general anaesthetic, so it should be painless. And it's done through your vagina, so there's no cutting of the skin. On the other hand, there is now some feeling that too many D and Cs are being done. By my calculation, very nearly half the women in Britain will end up having one – which does seem a bit excessive, to put it mildly!

So talk the operation over carefully with the surgeon, and make sure that it's necessary before you go ahead.

---

does rot your teeth!

Of course, nearly all of us enjoy a good meal of 'forbidden' foods now and again. And there's no doubt that a thoroughly wicked meal – with all the things you're not really supposed to eat – can be the prelude to a highly successful evening in bed.

Perhaps I should add that if you believe in *aphrodisiac* foods, then there's no harm at all in adding them to your diet. I have to say, however, that there's no medical evidence that champagne, oysters, *coquilles St. Jacques* or octopus actually work.

But the good thing about allegedly aphrodisiac foods is that if a person *believes* in them, then they'll do her or him some good. Also, if your dinner partner orders oysters and champagne, you do at least have some idea of what she or he has in mind!

DYSPAREUNIA

Dyspareunia

'Ye Gods,' I hear you say, 'What's dyspareunia? (And how do you pronounce it?)'

Well, it's pronounced 'diss-par-YEW-nya'. And it means 'pain on intercourse'. For some reason, the term dyspareunia is almost always applied to pain experienced by women.

Now, what can cause pain during intercourse?

The first group of physical causes are the common (all too common!) vaginal infections. These are: thrush (candida); trichomonas ('trich'); certain other infections, and, occasionally, herpes.

Clearly, the remedy for all these is to get yourself (and, if necessary, your partner) diagnosed and treated as soon as possible. (If you don't want to see your GP, you can call your local health authority for the address of your nearest Special Clinic.) Your local Well-Woman Clinic may also be able to help, although not all of them are able to prescribe treatment.

Non-infectious causes of intercourse pain include the following:

Urethral caruncle: a swelling occurring at the opening of the waterworks. Treatment: removal.

Endometriosis: an inflammatory condition of the internal organs; tends to cause *deep* pain on sex. Treatment: hormones or surgery.

Post-menopause vaginitis: tenderness caused by the drop in female hormones. Treatment: female hormones.

Post-episiotomy (or post-childbirth tear) pain: Lubricants such as KY, Durol or Senselle may help. If not, see a gynae expert.

Prolapsed ovary: if your ovary is lying too low in your pelvis, this can cause pain in some positions of intercourse. Treatment: choose another position.

Cervical erosion: at least one in ten women has an erosion of the

DYSPAREUNIA

cervix. This may occasionally cause deep dyspareunia. Treatment: usually cautery of the erosion.

Uncommonly in Britain, deep pain may be due to the chronic disability called pelvic inflammatory disease (PID). Very, very rarely, it may be due to cancer of the cervix.

Note that I have not listed a 'small vagina' as a physical cause of intercourse pain. Though many people still believe in the myth of the small vagina as a common reason for pain, I've not seen a single case since I qualified in 1962.

In fact, nearly all alleged cases of 'narrow vagina' turn out to be due to a fantastically common emotional problem called vaginismus, in which the pelvic muscles tighten up whenever an approach is made to the vagina. This can usually be cured or helped by relaxation therapy.

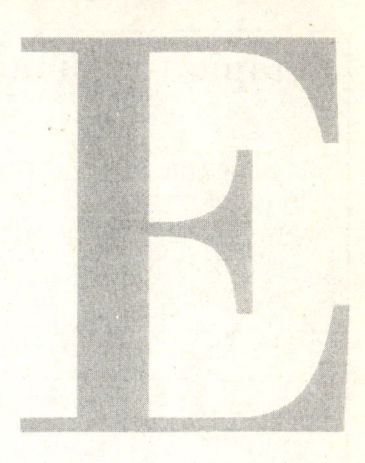

ECTOPIC PREGNANCY

Ectopic Pregnancy

This means pregnancy occurring outside the normal situation (i.e. the womb). In the great majority of such cases, the fertilised egg lodges in the Fallopian tube (which connects the ovary to the womb). Where this happens there is virtually no possibility that the baby can be born.

In fact, it usually becomes apparent that something is wrong not long after the first period is missed. The symptoms vary a good deal, but usually the woman experiences quite severe pain low down in the abdomen, on either the right or the left side, depending on which tube is involved. Sometimes the pain is accompanied by giddiness. Within a few hours there is usually vaginal bleeding.

In some cases of ectopic pregnancy there is severe bleeding inside the abdomen. If this happens, the patient collapses and is pale, shocked and gasping for breath. She *must* be got to hospital immediately.

The only treatment for ectopic pregnancy is to remove the foetus by surgical operation. Usually the Fallopian tube has to be taken away as well. This doesn't mean that the patient is now sterile, however; if the other tube is healthy, there is no reason why she should not have children in the future.

Ectopic pregnancies are probably commoner in women who are using the IUD – and possibly in women who are on the mini-Pill.

Q May I give a word of encouragement to your reader who wondered if she could have a baby after having an ectopic pregnancy? I had an ectopic, and was therefore left with only one tube. But afterwards, I was lucky enough to produce three children.

A Thank you very much, ma'am! Good of you to give this encouragement to the many women who've had ectopics.

Q I've had an ectopic pregnancy; as a result, one of my tubes was removed. We've been trying since then to start a family, but no luck. What are my chances?

ECTOPIC PREGNANCY • EXERCISE

A Perfectly all right – *if* your other tube is OK. If you've been trying unsuccessfully for over a year, then I think it's time you went to a gynaecologist to have a test to reveal whether this tube is bunged up or not.
Good luck.

Exercise

There's no doubt that sensible exercise benefits your general health. For that reason, a sensible amount of exercise is likely to benefit your sex life too – simply by toning up your body.

The widespread belief that exercise – and, in particular, jogging – will reduce your libido is nonsense! I keep encountering athletes who assure me that 'medical research' has proved that running makes you less sexy.

Well, the 'medical research' in question was an April Fool's Day joke published by my own medical journal, *General Practitioner*! We ran a completely bogus story – made up by a Buckinghamshire GP, Dr Bev Daily – about how a completely fictional American university had shown that exercise makes people lose their interest in sex because it raises the temperature in their running shorts!

This wonderfully daft story was swallowed hook, line and sinker by the London *Daily Mail*, and was duly published and flashed round the world. All our subsequent efforts to convince people that the story was a hoax have failed, and it's still quoted. If they were to look at the original article, they'd find that the give-away was a small paragraph near the end in which Dr Daily claimed that scientists were even now working on a device to combat 'exercise-induced loss of libido' – a pocket refrigerator to be worn inside the shorts!

In all this, however, there is one faint echo of truth. It's this: really *intensive* exercise over a long spell of time (the sort of thing that serious Olympic contenders engage in) does have an effect on women's sex glands – it takes their periods away. Indeed, I am reliably informed that the highly-trained women's athletics squads of most western nations have almost all of them lost their periods at one time or another.

FALLOPIAN TUBES

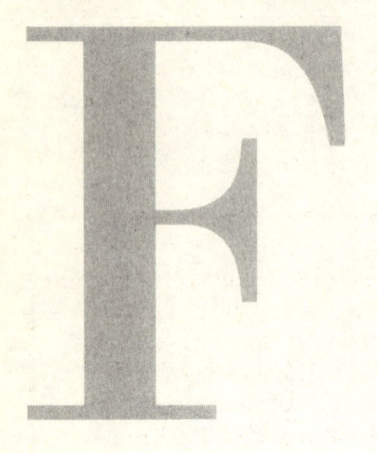

The Fallopian Tubes

Your 'tubes' are among the most vital organs of your body – vital to the human race that is. Why? Because until very recently, it was completely impossible for a baby to be born unless his or her mum had at least one healthy fallopian tube. And unfortunately, women's tubes are often far from healthy.

Fallopian tubes are the little bits of tubing which link your ovaries to your womb. You have a left tube and a right tube. Each one is about 4" (10cm) long. The outer end makes a sort of funnel shape which points towards your ovary, the idea being that when an egg is released from the ovary, it'll go into the funnel and find its way down the tube and into your womb.

It's thought that fertilisation usually takes place within the tube – in other words, that's where the sperm meets the egg. And once the egg's been fertilised, it tries to find a suitable place on the womb lining on which to implant.

The *inside* of the tube is extremely narrow, and it's lined with cells which project out into the tube like stalactites and stalagmites in a long, narrow cave.

FALLOPIAN TUBES

Blocked Tubes

A tremendously common cause of infertility in women is blocked tubes. If the Fallopian tubes are blocked for any reason, the man's sperm can't get through to the woman's ova.

The causes of this difficulty are:

a previous sterilization operation (some women undergo sterilization, then get divorced and remarried and want their tubes unblocked)

previous infection of the tubes;

inflammatory disorders in the lower abdomen – for instance, reaction to a past burst appendix, or endometriosis.

I have to say that tube blockage due to previous infection of the tubes is far more common than most people realise, and that these infections are often – though very far from always – sexually transmitted.

However, your tubes *can* become infected in other ways, for instance, as a result of using an IUD. I'm not suggesting that if you have blocked tubes, you should feel guilty about some affair of long ago.

How Do You Find Out Your Tubes Are Blocked?

If you have had serious difficulties in conceiving, then the infertility experts will usually want to investigate you for possible tube blockage. This *can't* be diagnosed by a simple vaginal examination. It has to be done by one of these means:

special X-rays of the tubes

injecting gas through the tubes to see if it goes through freely

laparoscopy.

How To Get Treated

Firstly, it may sometimes be possible to treat the underlying disease – for instance, if an infection is still present, to treat it with antibiotics. The common cause of tube blockage, endometriosis, can often be successfully treated with hormones or surgery (including laser surgery).

Secondly, a totally blocked tube can sometimes be repaired by delicate surgery, working with an operating microscope (microsurgery).

Thirdly, the 'test-tube baby' technique may be used to bypass the blockage altogether.

FERTILISATION

Fertilisation

I find it incredible that each of us is here because a single microscopic sperm met a single microscopic ovum in somebody's Fallopian tube. Or – in the case of test-tube babies – in somebody's laboratory.

That is, of course, what 'fertilisation' means – the union of a man's sperm with a woman's ovum (egg).

What happens is that when a couple make love, a living pool of sperm is deposited around the woman's cervix. It usually contains anything between 300 million and 500 million of the little 'tadpoles'.

Most of the fluid eventually runs out of the vagina. But a large number of the sperms streak upwards, through the cervix, through the womb, and into the Fallopian tubes, looking for a likely ovum to fertilise.

If the woman has just ovulated (this tends to happen at midcycle), just such an ovum will be innocently making its way down one of the Fallopian tubes.

The fastest and most determined of the sperms reaches her, penetrates her – and that's that! Some might say that there's an interesting analogy with male human behaviour here . . .

Fertilisation usually seems to take place in the outer third of a woman's Fallopian tube, but it could occur either higher up or lower down.

Unfortunately, if it occurs *too* high up (before the ovum has actually got into the funnel-like opening of the Fallopian tube) the result will probably be an ectopic – i.e. 'out of place' – pregnancy. This can hardly ever survive.

And if fertilisation occurs too low down (for instance, if the sperm and ovum meet in the womb) then again there's no chance that the fertilised ovum will live.

But if the woman and man have synchronised their lovemaking correctly so that the ripe ovum and the intrepid sperm meet in the right place, then the two of them will fuse together – and the resulting fertilised ovum will continue on its passage down the Fallopian tube and into the womb, where with luck it will 'implant' in the womb lining a few days later.

In practice, it does seem that a very high percentage of fertilised ova fail to implant in the lining of the womb. In these cases, the woman simply menstruates – and never even realises that her ovum was fertilised that month.

GARDNERELLA · GONORRHOEA

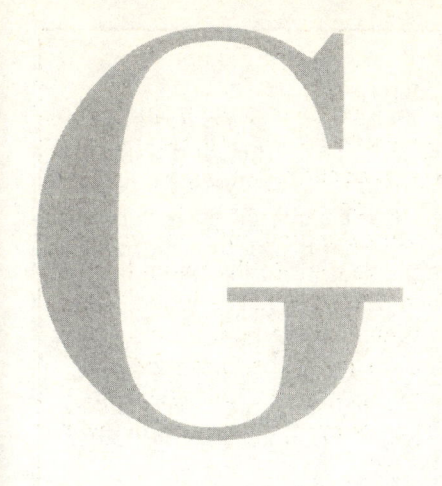

Gardnerella

This is a relatively newly discovered vaginal infection, but one which is increasingly commonly diagnosed, especially in the USA.

The chief symptom is a greyish vaginal discharge. Response to the drug metronidazole is good.

Gonorrhoea

This form of VD is regrettably still common in every country in the world. In men, gonorrhoea produces two dramatic symptoms, about two to five days after having sex with someone who is infected. These are: severe pain on passing water ('like passing razor blades'), and a copious discharge from the penis.

There can be other symptoms if you've taken part in oral or other forms of sex. And there can be very serious and painful complications later.

Fortunately, treatment with adequate doses of penicillin cures most people. But at all costs, don't sleep with anyone till you're cured. This kind of behaviour is almost criminally

GONORRHOEA

stupid – yet some men are thoughtless enough to do it.

The most tragic thing about gonorrhoea is that *in most women it produces no symptoms*. In some instances, there may be an episode of pain, fever or vaginal discharge. But in most cases, what happens is that the woman makes love with somebody (perhaps someone she has a holiday romance with), becomes infected, but *doesn't realise*.

For months or even years thereafter, the gonorrhoea germ may be damaging her health – and specifically the health of her pelvic organs. It may make her sterile, or give her salpingitis.

Fortunately, many women *do* have their cases diagnosed – because the infection is detected in their partner and he tells them that they need treatment.

So, if you ever feel that you have 'taken a risk' get a full confidential check-up – preferably at a specialist Genito-Urinary Clinic of the type available in Britain and some other countries.

Once gonorrhoea has been successfully diagnosed it can be treated – usually very successfully, if it's caught early enough. Treatment is usually with penicillin.

Penicillin-resistant gonorrhoea can usually be defeated by other drugs, such as spectinomycin.

Finally, here are a few tips for avoiding gonorrhoea and other types of VD:

avoid casual sex and one-night stands

consider using a barrier method of contraception – it helps a bit

be wary of dates with men who are air travellers – international travellers have been shown to be particularly liable to acquire and spread VD (often the resistant kind)

if in doubt after a sexual contact, always have an internal check-up.

HERPES

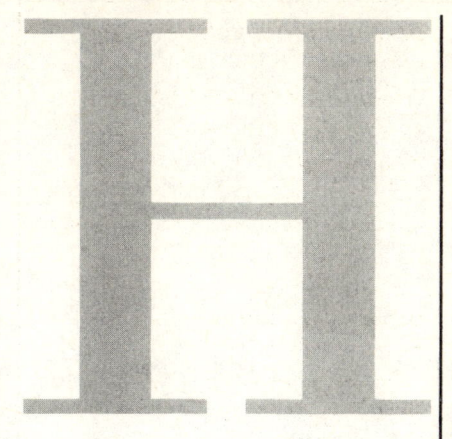

Q I would kill myself if it weren't for the fact that I have a child to support. After 15 years of faithful but not very happy marriage, I separated from my husband last year.

For a while after that I had the most fantastic time. I hadn't realised that men would find me so attractive. I had four lovers in a row — and sex with them was wonderful (far better than it was with my husband). It was beautiful to find that I could go on for hours and hours. I was very happy.

Then it happened: I got herpes. I understand that there is nothing that can be done, and that I can never make love again.

A No, that isn't true. I happen to know the very well-qualified doctor who is treating you, and if you go and see him again he will tell you (a) that herpes often does burn itself out; (b) that new drugs are giving promising results; and (c) that a cure will probably be found eventually. Good luck.

Q I am faithful to my boyfriend, and he has been faithful to me.

But four months ago, I developed small blisters at the opening of my

HERPES

vagina. The clinic was very nice, but told me it was herpes.

I felt so ashamed that I never mentioned it to anyone, not even my boyfriend.

But as the attack of herpes was really very mild, is there a chance it won't come back?

A Yes, this is possible. But the odds are that you may get further attacks. If so, let's hope they're mild ones again.

What worries me is that you haven't told your boyfriend! Presumably you acquired the herpes virus from him — or perhaps you got it from a previous lover. If the latter is true, then you may have infected your boyfriend too.

So I feel the most honest thing to do would be to tell him the truth — and to go back together to the Genito-Urinary Clinic ('Special Clinic') for mutual counselling.

Q Sometimes my fiancé develops minute blister-like lesions on his penis. And I sometimes experience a severe burning sensation after passing water. Could this be serious?

A I have to be frank and say that there's a chance this could be herpes. (But as I've said before, herpes isn't as big a reason for panic as the newspapers seem to think.)

Anyway, both of you should definitely go to a 'special clinic' for a confidential check-up.

Q Is it true that there's some sort of organisation for people who have had herpes?

A Yes, write to the Herpes Association c/o *Spare Rib*, 27 Clerkenwell Close, London EC1 0AT.

Q I have definitely contracted vaginal herpes as a direct result of having oral sex when my partner had a cold sore on his mouth.

I feel strongly that you should immediately advise everybody not to participate in oral sex while suffering from an outbreak of cold sores.

A I do agree. In fact, I have long advised against having oral love play whilst people are suffering from *any* kind of mouth or throat infection.

The virus which causes the common 'cold sore' on the lip is so similar to the virus of genital herpes

HERPES

that it may eventually transpire that the current outbreak of genital herpes in the USA and Britain is linked with the fact that oral sex has become so popular in the last two decades or so.

I'm sorry to hear about your herpes, and hope you succeed in defeating it.

Q I am getting very bad menopause symptoms. Would hormone therapy be the answer?

A Hormone replacement therapy (HRT) helps most women with

Herpes

So many people are worried about herpes; however, the statistical chance of catching it in Britain (in contrast to the USA) is still low, with only about 12,000 reported cases a year.

But everybody ought to know the classic symptoms. These include painful little blisters on the sex organs – rather like the 'cold sores' so many people get on their mouths. (In fact, the virus which causes cold sores is very closely related to the one which causes herpes.) There can be many other symptoms, including itching, inability to pass water, fever, headache and muscle pains. But it's the blisters you should look out for.

If you think you've got herpes, you should get yourself to a *Sexually Transmitted Disease clinic*

as fast as possible. There's still no actual cure for the infection, but the drug acyclovir (Zovirax) relieves symptoms and reduces the duration of attacks. There is a vaccine, but it doesn't seem to work. Press reports of a 'cure' invented by 'Dr' Stephan (of the so-called 'Harley St Hit-Man' case) are nonsense: Mr Stephan isn't really a doctor, and does not have a cure for herpes.

But let me finish with one piece of relatively good news. Most members of the public seem to be convinced that 'Herpes is forever'. This is now known to be untrue. Many people only have one single attack, and there is a definite tendency for the disease to burn itself out. So if you've got herpes, please *don't* despair.

HORMONE REPLACEMENT

menopause symptoms – but nothing is 100% certain in medicine, and I can't promise that you'd be helped.

However, if I were a woman with severe 'change of life' symptoms I think that I'd unhesitatingly take the hormones for a spell – provided that they were given under careful supervision, with regular health checks. Good luck.

Q I'm a woman of 47 and I am really desperate because the hormone treatment which I'm having for the menopause isn't helping my appalling baldness. I am even losing possible jobs because of my appearance. NHS wigs look awful and I'm short of money for a top-class one.

A I'm sorry to hear about this. You are seeing one of the most famous endocrinologists in the country, and you should ask him whether there is any hope at all that the baldness will get better. If the answer's 'no' then I think you could try one of the following: a good class wig, a hair transplant, or hair 'weaving'. I'm afraid all of these are very expensive. But since your baldness is having such a disastrous effect on your employment prospects, I'm sure that any bank manager would be willing to give you a long-term loan to cover the cost. Good luck.

Q I have just reached the menopause, and my doctor has put me on hormone replacement therapy for hot flushes. What I want to know is, do I need to go on

Hygiene

First things first. How do you keep the intimate, sexual places of your body in the best possible trim?

Whether you are a man or a woman, a daily wash of the genital organs in hand-hot water with mild soap is a must. You don't actually need to have a bath every day of your life, though of course many people find it invigorating and refreshing.

Too *many* baths can in fact be bad for the sex organs. Many women, and some men, find that they keep getting irritating attacks of thrush and other fungus infections if they have too many hot baths. If *you* have any tendency to thrush or to those trying fungal infections of the skin between the thighs, you would almost certainly do better to have cool showers than hot tubs.

HYGIENE

taking it for the rest of my life?

I feel that if I don't go on taking it, by the time I'm 55, I'll be looking like Phil Collins instead of Joan Collins!

A You will need it until you find that when you have a break, the hot flushes don't come back. But you can take it for longer (indeed, for ten or 20 years), if your doc agrees, and if you feel it's doing you good.

There are risks from 'HRT', but some gynaecologists now think women should take it for life to avoid osteoporosis (brittle bone disease).

Whether you are female or male, *avoid* applying chemical agents to your genital area. Be especially wary if you have sensitive skin or are prone to allergic reactions. Even bubble baths can sometimes be harmful to those delicate tissues!

Because men's genitals are less complicated, they have less to worry about where health and hygiene are concerned. However, a man *does* have to keep his genitals in reasonable hygienic trim, for three reasons:

if you don't observe the simple rules of hygiene described below, you increase your chances of cancer of the penis.

men who aren't hygienic tend to give their sexual partners certain illnesses — including, possibly, cancer of the cervix

unless you keep yourself clean 'down below', you're likely to discover that women find you, to say the least, unappealing, especially where oral sex is concerned!

Some readers may find it incredible that it's necessary to tell the above facts to any man. But I do assure you that doctors find that a distressing proportion of the men whom they have to examine have simply *no* idea of personal genital hygiene at all. (Yuk!)

All males should wash their genitals at least once a day, paying special attention to the part of the male organ just below the 'head' — this is where the skin glands produce a material called 'smegma', which rapidly accumulates in unhygienic males.

If the man isn't circumcised, he should take care to draw his foreskin back before washing.

Hysterectomy

An incredible one in five of all women have this operation at some stage in their lives, so it's well worth your while knowing exactly what it involves. Hysterectomy just means removal of the womb or uterus, and nothing else.

Because few people understand anatomy, they tend to get confused about hysterectomy in two ways. Firstly, they often think that the operation involves taking away all or part of the vagina and will therefore make it impossible for the woman to have intercourse ever again. This is nonsense.

No part of the vagina is removed. When the womb has been taken out, this leaves a little gap at the very top of the vagina, and that gap is sewn up by the surgeon.

Some gynaecologists say that this actually makes the vagina a bit longer than it was before. Anyway, it certainly isn't any smaller, so it'll be just as effective a love-making organ as ever it was. Once the stitches at the very top of the vagina have healed, you'll be able to resume love-making just as before.

Some women find that their climaxes feel a little different because the womb has gone. Many women enjoy sex more than they did before for two reasons: whatever womb condition they were suffering from has been cured, and now that the womb has been removed, the fear of unwanted pregnancy is gone forever.

A second source of confusion is the muddle in people's minds over the womb and the ovaries. Many women (and men) think that if you have a hysterectomy this will stop your output of female hormones: they believe that you will therefore get hot flushes, put on weight, become neurotic and goodness only knows what else besides. Once again, this is utter nonsense. It is the ovaries, not the womb, which produce female hormones. *As long as the ovaries aren't removed at the same time*, your hysterectomy won't produce any of the distressing symptoms of hormone deficiency.

HYSTERECTOMY

Removal of the Ovaries

Regrettably, it is sometimes necessary to remove the ovaries at the same time as a hysterectomy is done, though this only happens in a minority of cases. The ovaries may have to be taken out because they contain cysts or because they're diseased.

If the surgeon removes them while you're still young (indeed, at any stage before the change of life), then I'm afraid that there's every chance that the resulting sharp drop in hormones will give you quite severe menopausal symptoms in the days after the operation – mainly in the form of hot flushes and sweating attacks. There may also be vaginal dryness later on.

Fortunately, however, these distressing symptoms can be prevented with carefully prescribed doses of female hormones over the next few months or even years. But make sure you get the treatment: a disquieting number of younger women complain that they were never offered it.

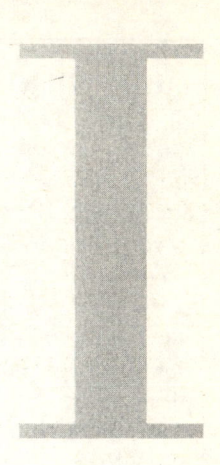

IMPLANTATION · IMPOTENCE

Implantation

What is implantation? Well, it's the process whereby a fertilised egg (ovum) becomes embedded in your womb.

Fertilisation — which is the union of a sperm with your ovum — normally takes place in the outer part of one of your Fallopian tubes.

But that doesn't necessarily mean that you're going to get pregnant. The fertilised ovum has quite a way to go before it embeds itself in your womb lining and starts to put down roots into it. That's implantation.

The fertilised ovum is impossible to see with the naked eye. It makes its way through the long cavern of your Fallopian tube, emerges into the uterus, and then may or may not find a suitable spot on the womb lining in which to embed itself.

If it doesn't find a suitable spot, then that particular ovum will be lost — and you won't become pregnant that month. This often happens.

The journey from the point of fertilisation down to the point of implantation takes quite a time — it's thought to be five to seven days in most cases. Implantation doesn't occur till nearly a week after you made love.

That time gap of five to seven days is of tremendous practical and philosophical importance these days. Why? Because it's on that time gap that the whole principle of the 'Morning After Pill' and the 'Morning After Coil' is based.

You see, many doctors now feel that it is not wrong to pre-

Q I notice you often recommend Family Planning Clinics as a source of help for sex problems. I took my impotent husband to one near us, but they didn't want to know.

A Oh dear. Not all Family Planning Clinics provide 'Balint treatment' — a form of brief psychotherapy/counselling which helps many men and women with sex problems. The cuts of recent years have had a disastrous effect on clinic services in many areas.

So here are two alternative sources of help and counselling for your husband. Send a large s.a.e., to either of these two organisations, asking for the name of their nearest available therapists to: The

IMPOTENCE

vent pregnancy by giving a special pill (or fitting an IUD) between the time of fertilisation and the time of implantation.

Others feel that it *is* wrong, and that to do it is to take life.

Certainly, the fertilised ovum is living (as, indeed, are the sperms and the unfertilised ovum). But a world authority on conception and contraception, Dr John Guillebaud says that as a Christian doctor he feels that pregnancy is not established till implantation has taken place – and that therefore it is not immoral to prevent that implantation.

The philosophical issues are very complex. But the law certainly makes no objection to the use of 'Morning-After' methods in order to prevent implantation.

Institute of Psycho-Sexual Medicine, *11 Chandos Street, London W1M 9DE*; The Association of Sexual and Marital Therapists, *PO Box 62, Sheffield S10 3TS*. Good luck.

Q In our 31-year marriage my husband has had intercourse with me exactly three times. I have spent my married life crying myself to sleep because of this. But we have never, ever discussed it. Only now (when I have reached the menopause) have I broken down in tears in front of him. But I suppose it's too late to do anything now?

A Not necessarily, ma'am. Your long and sad letter suggests that your husband has a considerable impotence problem. But if your GP sent the pair of you to a sex therapist, it could be sorted out.

And even if it couldn't, the therapist could still guide you both to loving and gentle ways of obtaining mutual fulfilment. Good luck to you.

Impotence

The American sex researchers, Masters and Johnson claimed impotence to affect 40% of American marriages to some extent, and the same *might* possibly be true of other countries, though figures are lacking. Certainly, the problem's a very widespread one.

Many cases of impotence are thought by doctors to be psychological in origin. Among the exceptions are impotence associated with diabetes and blood-vessel disease, and

IMPOTENCE • INCONTINENCE

impotence caused by drugs, *e.g.* tablets for high blood pressure, and alcohol.

Most patients find difficulty in accepting that their problems could be due to stress, tiredness or emotional hang-ups, and willingly ascribe their impotence to such improbable causes as hormone or vitamin deficiency, or to advancing age. They may fall into the clutches of quacks, and spend a good deal of money on useless but expensive 'tonics', 'rejuvenatives', and 'aphrodisiacs'.

Unfortunately, the impotent patient who goes to his doctor may not always obtain a great deal of help, for several reasons. In the first place, as a medical journal grimly remarked recently, 'the doctor may be in the same boat himself'. Regrettably, a doctor's training doesn't usually include much formal teaching on sexual problems, and it is unfortunately true that many middle-aged men are erroneously told that their impotence is due to their age. In fact, age is no bar to sexual performance: many men are quite potent at 80 or even 90!

There is no short and easy answer to the problem of impotence. Patients will often demand hormone tablets or injections from their doctors, before eventually discovering that no magic 'instant remedy' exists.

What *can* be done about impotence then? Where there's no *physical* cause, the patient and his partner should learn to accept the fact that his problem

---

Q My mother, aged 77, is very fit and still rides a bike. But her problem is that she is often very incontinent of urine. I suppose it's old and weak muscles, is it?

A Yes, it's a similar problem to the 'lax pelvic floor' one. But your mum's symptoms are so severe that she really ought to consult a gynaecologist – to see whether a 'tightening-up' op is what's needed.

Q I am a nurse, and pregnant. I know that my husband's seminal fluid contains prostaglandins, and remember learning that these can induce labour. Could I use

INDUCED LABOUR

is an understandable emotional one. When this is done, and he recognises that he is not suffering from either some horrible disease or from 'lack of manhood', the problem is then cut down to size and becomes simply a matter of overcoming his own sexual repressions and anxieties or tiredness!

A surprising number of men will achieve this victory over a period of time, sometimes aided by rest, a change of job, or anti-depressants. For others, however, recovery may be very difficult, even with the help of a loving and understanding wife. A 'second honeymoon' together, away from children and the stress of work, may be of considerable value.

The most effective therapy available is the 'sexual retraining' developed in the USA by Masters and Johnson. But in Britain the impotent man and his wife will derive very considerable benefits from learning similar techniques to those of Masters and Johnson taught at many National Marriage Guidance Council centres ('Relate') and Family Planning Clinics.

Happily, the last few years have seen major improvements in the treatment of the type of impotence that is due to physical causes. Urological surgeons can now insert 'splints' (including inflatable splints) into the penis. They can also prescribe injections, which can be given directly into the penis in order to produce an immediate erection.

---

sex as a way of starting labour?

Also, when I reach a climax during pregnancy, what effect does it have on the baby?

A Remarkably little research has been done on the effect of maternal climax during pregnancy. I know of no evidence that it does the baby any harm.

Male sex fluid does contain the chemicals called prostaglandins, and these compounds can induce labour (knowledge based on the discovery of the rather yukky practice of a remote African tribe – who use an *oral* draught of semen to induce labour).

I'm open to correction, but I doubt whether having ordinary intercourse would deliver enough prostaglandins to the area of the uterus to make you go into labour.

IUD

Q My doctor has recommended a coil for me. But I'm not married, and I thought that it was contra-indicated for single women?

A Well, the intra-uterine device (IUD) is fine for most women *who have had children*.

The smaller types of IUD can easily be fitted in women who've never been pregnant. But the risk of side-effects (such as infection) does seem to be quite high – particularly if the person has several lovers.

I do not say that you *mustn't* have an IUD. But I do reckon you should get a second opinion from a Family Planning Clinic first.

Q I am 21 and have only recently starting having sex. Would the IUD be a good method for me to choose, as one of my friends has suggested?

A Doctors are now increasingly wary about fitting intra-uterine devices into 'nullips' – that is, women who've never been pregnant.

This is mainly because the risks of pelvic infection seem to be considerably higher in this group. No one knows why this should be. But it's been suggested that one factor may be that single women tend to have multiple partners.

Pelvic infection can have disastrous effects on your health and fertility. (For instance, it may block your tubes.) So think very carefully indeed before you agree to have an IUD.

Q I have had a coil for some time, and it was fine to begin with. But suddenly I've starting having periods that are two weeks long. Why?

A It's normal for periods to be longer on the coil and other types of IUD – but not as long as this.

When a woman who's using an IUD suddenly starts getting very long or painful periods, there must be some cause. *Very often, the device has started to come out.*

So get yourself a check-up from a GP or family planning clinic soonest – meantime, avoid sex as you may be at risk of pregnancy if the coil is coming out.

Q I am 23 and have just lost my virginity. Would you recommend that I use the IUD as a contraceptive?

214

IUD

A Well, congratulations on holding out till 23 – a major achievement these days!

Though the IUD (loop or coil, or whatever you like to call it) can be a wonderful method of contraception for some, it's important for women to realise that it may occasionally have disastrous side-effects. *And these side-effects are much more likely to happen in women who – like yourself – have never been pregnant.* One of the major risks in a 'never pregnant' woman is that of infection, possibly in part because many unmarried women have more than one lover.

If the infection gets to your tubes, it can make you sterile. So talk things over *very* carefully with your GP or family planning clinic before you elect to use an IUD.

Q I was fitted with some sort of IUD which was shaped like the figure '7'. Not long afterwards, I got a severe infection in my tube, and spent two weeks in hospital. Could the infection have been connected with the coil?

A Yes – though you might have trouble proving a 'cause-and-effect' relationship. But, as I've been saying in this column for years, pelvic infections are more common in women who use any type of IUD – including the now-famous Dalkon Shield.

Q My doctor said I could have an IUCD, but the clinic have offered me an IUD instead. What's the difference?

A There isn't any difference. People get a bit confused about this because of the fact that some doctors say 'IUD' (meaning 'intra-uterine device') while others say 'IUCD' (meaning 'intra-uterine *contraceptive* device').

There's no truth in the rumour that the letters 'IUD' stand for 'It's up dere!'

Make sure you understand about possible side-effects before you have an IUD (see previous question).

The IUD

'IUD' stands for 'intra-uterine device'. This description covers all of the many devices which are placed inside the womb, including the coil, the famous

IUD

Lippes loop, and the various copper devices.

Many millions of women world-wide rely on the IUD for protection against unwanted pregnancy. In the USA, however, its popularity has been limited by the sad occurrence of a number of disastrous infections in women who were using a brand called the Dalkon Shield.

That particular brand of IUD has long been taken off the market, but it must be admitted that there is a small danger of womb and tube infection with any type of IUD. Bear in mind that if the tube infection does occur and is left untreated, this could seriously affect your future fertility.

But the *common* side-effects of IUDs are:

heavy periods

prolonged periods

expulsion of the device.

Despite these and other much rarer side-effects, IUDs suit four out of every five women who try them. The insertion process takes only a few minutes; it's generally much easier and less uncomfortable if the woman has had children.

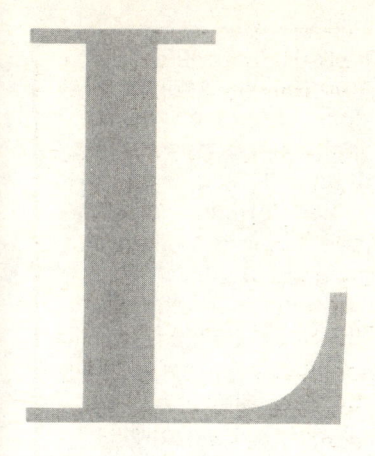

LACTATION

Lactation

Lactation really is the most amazing function. Despite the fact that breast-feeding temporarily became rather unpopular in the late 20th century, it's true that the vast majority of human beings who've ever lived have owed their survival to the fact that their mums lactated.

How does it all work? The interior of your breast is rather like a bunch of grapes. The milk is manufactured in those little sacs, and then it comes down a series of ducts into the reservoirs – between 15 and 20 little chambers which lie right behind your nipple.

During pregnancy, the sacs are stimulated by female hormones to grow and to get ready to produce milk. Some authorities reckon that this process makes the average woman add three pounds to the weight of her bosom during pregnancy. (Certainly, the late and much-missed Diana Dors used to say that becoming pregnant was the only way she knew for a woman to significantly increase the size of her bust.)

Small amounts of fluid may be secreted in late pregnancy, but it's not until you've been delivered of the afterbirth (placenta)

LACTATION

that things really start happening. The placenta is a rich source of hormones, and the moment it's gone there's a remarkable 'all change' in the hormonal balance of your body.

In particular, the front part of your pituitary gland releases a hormone called prolactin to start stimulating those milk sacs to produce.

However, lactation probably *won't* go very well unless you're given the chance to put your baby to the breast, and let her/him suck firmly and frequently. It is suckling your baby which actually stimulates the pituitary gland (at the base of your brain) to produce both prolactin and – very importantly – oxytocin.

Oxytocin is another pituitary hormone. It works on the ducts so that the milk 'comes on down' – the rather startling sensation described by many women as 'my milk coming in'.

I can't really over-emphasise the fact that unless the breast is regularly suckled, your pituitary won't be stimulated – and therefore lactation will probably fail. That's why birth expert Sheila Kitzinger says that 'love play involving playing with the breasts and sucking and stimulating them is probably the best preparation for breast-feeding.'

MASTECTOMY

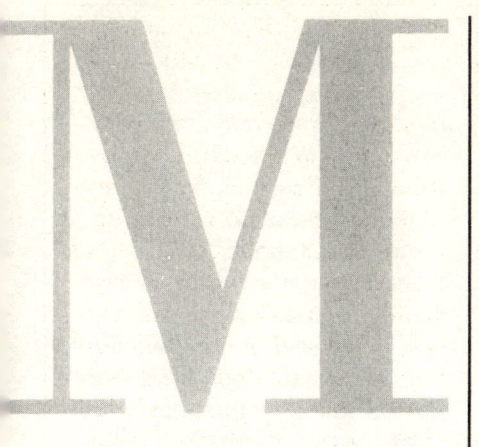

Q My wife is devastated by the fact that she has just had a breast removed.

She cannot believe that I still desire her. How can I convince her that this is so?

A Well sir, unfortunately many women do find it very hard to believe they are still loved and desired after losing a breast.

Ideally, ladies should have careful pre-operative emotional counselling before a mastectomy operation – but this doesn't seem to have happened in your wife's case.

So, I urge you to call on the services of that marvellous organisation, the Breast Care and Mastectomy Association; their counsellors and their literature may well help her. Write to them (enclosing sae) at: *26A Harrison Street, London WC1H 8JG.*

Meantime, all you can do is keep telling her that you love and want her very much.

THE MENOPAUSE

The Menopause

Let's get the blokes out of the way first. *There is no such thing as a menopause in men.* After all, 'menopause' actually means 'cessation of the periods' — and I need hardly remind you that men don't actually *have* periods! The various symptoms which people are all too ready to attribute to a 'male menopause' are actually due to such causes as psychological stress and overwork — *not* to hormonal changes. For men, unlike women, are very fortunate in that the output of their sex hormones falls only very, very slowly over a period of 20 to 30 years from the 40s onwards.

Women, however, are different in that their sex hormone output falls very rapidly indeed at the time of the menopause (average age 49 in Britain). This can result in very trying symptoms.

All I need stress here is that the menopause does NOT mean the end of your sex life, or of your physical attractiveness or womanly beauty. You may not even get any 'menopausal' symptoms — like hot flushes — but if you do, these can usually be treated fairly successfully nowadays with hormone replacement therapy.

The menopause can be a blooming *awful* time for many women, but others sail through it without difficulty. A sympathetic and understanding husband and family can do much to alleviate the stresses and strains of the change of life. However, it's a PHYSICAL and not an 'emotional' one, so don't let anyone tell you different! Commonest symptoms are hot flushes, sweating attacks, and vaginal dryness.

Sex life, incidentally, should not be adversely affected by the menopause. In fact, many women find that once they are free of the nuisance of periods and (not long afterwards) free of the risk of unwanted pregnancy, life takes on the quality of a 'second honeymoon'.

How Should Periods Stop?

Most women are confused about this important point, and a lot of them think that heavy bleeding ('flooding'), or irregular bleeding is normal at this time. *This is a dangerous myth.*

There are only three ways in which the menopause should occur.
(1) periods stop suddenly and never return: or,

THE MENOPAUSE

(2) they get less and less in volume until they cease altogether; or,

(3) they get farther and farther apart in time until they stop completely.

Bleeding between the periods or after intercourse, irregular bleeding, or very heavy bleeding are all abnormal. If you have these symptoms, consult your doctor, who'll probably do an internal examination. He may then send you to a gynaecologist for further tests.

Of course, the cause of the trouble may be something relatively minor, like fibroids or an erosion of the cervix, but only proper investigation will tell whether this is the case. The risk of cancer of the womb and of the cervix is so great at this age that it is essential for you to consult your doctor at the least suspicion of anything being wrong.

Bleeding *after* the menopause is also a potentially serious symptom – if it occurs, see your doctor as soon as you can.

Menopausal Problems

Menopausal problems affect hundreds of thousands of women – and can mess up their sex lives. However, the outlook for your love-life is generally good – mainly because this is in some ways the very sexiest time of your life. (It's widely reckoned that women reach the peak of their sexual performance when they're over 40.)

Common menopausal problems are:

hot flushes (referred to in the USA as 'hot flashes')

sweating attacks

dryness of the vagina.

All of these are due to a relatively sudden drop in hormone levels. *And all of them can be successfully treated by hormone replacement therapy (HRT) using female hormones.*

The hormones can be given by mouth or by implant under the skin. However, where the main problem is a dry, sore vagina which is making intercourse difficult, it's a widespread practice to give the woman a tube of vaginal hormone cream.

A few weeks of nightly application of this will usually restore her vagina to its previous healthy state – and love-making to normal.

THE MENOPAUSE • MENSTRUATION

There's a very slight danger that her partner will absorb some of the hormone through the skin of his penis. A few men have temporarily developed little breasts as a result of this unusual method of absorption, but the risk is pretty small (like the breasts).

Oral female hormone dosage should be very carefully controlled by your own family doctor, gynaecologist or menopause clinic. It is believed that, in the past, overuse of unbalanced hormone preparations (particularly in the USA) has led to cases of cancer of the lining of the womb.

But, quite obviously, management of menopause symptoms is *not* simply a question of replacing a few hormones. All women who have menopausal problems need love and understanding from their husbands, families and friends.

Note: If you're having trouble getting hormone replacement therapy (HRT) or regular check-ups, contact the Family Planning Information Service (01-636 7866), who will tell you the address of the nearest Menopause Clinic.

Menstruation

Nearly all women menstruate — as a rule, between the ages of about 12 and 49. A woman menstruates on average 13 times a year, so she has to put up with something like 480 periods during her lifetime.

A woman's first few periods are often painless. But once she has menstruated a few times, the odds are that she will get at least some pain. It's thought that at least five million women in Britain, and at least 25 million in America, suffer from some degree of period pain (or 'dysmenorrhoea', to give it its posh name).

It's also important to realise that at least a fifth of that number suffer from menstruation which is *too heavy* or *too prolonged*. This is why so many women (in contrast to men) become anaemic: they lose too much iron in heavy or prolonged periods, so that the blood becomes weak.

Happily, modern treatment *can* help a woman combat painful, heavy or prolonged periods. In particular, I have to say that the fact that there are countless millions of women on the Pill has made a great difference to the world-wide problem of period

MENSTRUATION · MICTURITION

pain and appallingly heavy periods. Despite its possible side-effects, the Pill is remarkably good at:

abolishing period pain

lightening the menstrual flow

shortening the duration of menstruation.

But in view of the fact that menstruation causes women so many problems (you can't blame them for calling it 'the curse'!), you may ask why on earth a woman has to be bothered with it all. The reason is fairly straightforward. Each month, the womb builds up a rich lining, ready to receive a fertilised egg. This lining is filled with blood vessels. However, if *no* fertilised egg embeds itself in that rich lining (in other words, if the woman doesn't get pregnant that month), then her body's hormone balance 'tips' in such a way that the lining breaks up.

The break-up of the blood-rich lining naturally causes bleeding, and that's the period. The reason it looks a bit different from 'ordinary' blood is that it's mixed with debris and secretions from the womb lining.

Micturition

One function about which there's still considerable embarrassment is micturition. Even today, a lot of women (and indeed men) find it difficult to discuss the subject with their doctors — partly because they don't know any 'polite' term for having a pee.

Anyway, in an attempt to reduce the general embarrassment about this subject, let me explain just how micturition works. You have a urinary bladder which is located just in front of the upper part of your vagina. It's filled by two tubes (the ureters) which come down from your kidneys. And when it empties, the urine passes out through the short tube called the urethra.

At the outlet of the bladder, there are two tight constricting rings of muscle (called the sphincters) which prevent the urine from coming out till you want it to.

Normally, you are quite unaware of any sensation in your bladder until about 150ml of urine has accumulated in it (that's a little over a quarter of a pint).

At that stage, the nerves which run upwards from your

MICTURITION • MISCARRIAGE

bladder to your spinal cord and brain start sending a few mild signals – saying something like 'Listen, owner: we're going to have to do something about this in the next hour or two.'

But if more and more urine begins to accumulate in your bladder, you begin to feel discomfort. When the quantity reaches 600ml (which is a bit over a pint) the signals coming upwards become very urgent. If you tried to 'hold out' much longer you simply wouldn't be able to. Curiously enough, in pregnancy a woman *can* hold out much longer – the pregnant woman seems to have a sort of dispensation so that her bladder can hold at least twice as much.

When you finally decide that it's time to go to the loo, what happens is this.

One set of nerves relaxes the outer sphincter. Another set relaxes the inner sphincter – and makes your bladder contract. And that's it – you 'go'.

Finally, what *should* you say to your doc when you want to describe this important function? I would recommend either 'pass water' or 'pee'.

Q I have just suffered a miscarriage. Is there any way I could find out *why*?

A I'm so sorry to hear about this, as I'm sure it was distressing for you.

If it's any consolation, you're not alone: the recent *Delvin Report* suggested that almost one in five SHE readers have had 'a miss'.

In fact, about 20% of all pregnancies are thought to end in miscarriage. Usually the cause is totally unknown. So unless your doc has any suggestions, I think you may just have to write it off as upsetting but far from unusual.

Q This afternoon, my fiancé and I made love, and the condom split. After the tears and despairing laughter, we decided to go to my GP to ask for the 'morning after pill'.

My usual doctor wasn't free, so I had to see another one. To my indignation, she wouldn't give me the 'morning after pill' as it was against her religious beliefs about abortion!

Surely she has no right to mess about with my life in this way? Doctors aren't allowed to express their opinions like this, are they?

A I'm afraid that everybody is

MORNING AFTER PILL

Nentitled to express their views – and that nobody can force a doctor to do something which is against their ethical or religious principles.

However, while I respect this doctor's views, it does strike me as quite extraordinary to equate giving a pill (about two hours after sex) with abortion.

Your letter indicates that you were planning to see your regular GP the following day, and I hope you did so and got the tablets.

Nowadays, all GPs have the facility to prescribe the 'morning after pill', and most are willing to do so. It's just a question of taking two tablets of something called Schering PC4 – and then two more in 12 hours' time.

THE NIPPLE

Q I'm worried about the pink, circular area round my nipples.

This area is quite large, but when I'm cold and my nipples stick out, the pink disc shrivels up and looks really tiny.

I've never let any of my boyfriends see my breasts, because I feel so ashamed.

A No need for shame. The pigmented area round the nipple is *supposed* to shrivel up tightly when it's cold. So you're normal.

If you visit any of our chilly British nudist beaches this summer, you'll see that most of the women there have very small, retracted areolas. (And the chaps have their little problems with the cold, too . . .)

The Nipple

The nipple is one of the most sexually sensitive areas of the body – in both women *and* men. Some women can reach a climax through having just their nipples stimulated, though I don't know of any gents who can manage the same.

Anyway, let's get clear the basic anatomy of the nipple. Most people use the word wrongly: they think it means the *whole* of the pigmented disc in the middle of the breast. In fact, only the central bit which sticks out is called the nipple; the disc which surrounds it is called the areola.

The areola is quite sensitive too, but it doesn't have anywhere near as many nerve-endings as the actual nipple. The areola may be pink, brown or black – depending on your general colouring. It can be anything up to five inches (12.5cm) across, and there's no 'normal' size. People are sometimes worried by the little blobs which often run round the areola, but these are perfectly normal structures called 'the tubercles of Montgomery' (no connection with the Field-Marshal, as far as I know).

The nipple itself contains the openings of the 15–20 milk ducts, plus the aforementioned nerve endings – which are directly connected to one of the most important emotional regions of your brain. That's one reason why suckling a baby *and* sexual stimulation of the nipple both tend to have an immediate emotional impact on a woman.

The nipple also contains a lot

THE NIPPLE

Q Though I have large breasts, I have flat and underdeveloped nipples. Is there anything at all that I can do? I feel I am abnormal.

A Sorry to hear about this. The very latest results of *The Delvin Report* (our sex survey among 6,000 SHE readers) show that no less than 27% of respondents were unhappy about their breasts or nipples! However, *personally*, I reckon that if more women went to topless beaches and saw how other ladies are built 'up top', they'd be happier and realise that their bodies are *not* abnormal.

I do appreciate that you feel particularly badly about the flat-

of erectile tissue; in other words it can stand up, like a man's penis. Usually, both the nipple and the areola become much more prominent well before orgasm — but your areola loses its swelling very rapidly after a climax; the nipple usually takes quite a lot longer to go down.

Disorders

Inturning (inversion) of a nipple is common, and is *not* a disorder if you've had it all your adult life. If it makes breast-feeding difficult, then your midwife can prescribe you a 'nipple shell', which may help. But a sudden and unexplained inturning of the nipple *is* a potentially dangerous symptom, as it may indicate that a growth is pulling the nipple inwards. An urgent medical check is necessary.

Similarly, blood (or a brown discharge) coming from the nipple can be a danger sign. However, with luck it may only indicate a small papilloma (benign swelling) in a milk duct.

Finally (and I'm sorry to conclude on a gloomy note, but it is a very important one), a raw or weepy eczema-like patch on the nipple or areola in the over-45s must also be investigated *fast*, since it may indicate a malignant disorder called Paget's disease of the nipple. This has no connection with the more famous Paget's disease of bone, which is *not* malignant — Sir James Paget (1814–1899) confused everybody by being the first to describe at least four different diseases.

THE NIPPLE • NSU

ness of your nipples. If you really want to have something done about them, then it would be possible to have them 'elevated' by a plastic surgeon – though I don't believe that you could ever get this done on the Health Service. Good luck.

Q I have 'inverted nipples' and would like to get them sorted out before I go topless sunbathing this summer. Is it possible to have them corrected by operation?

A Yes, ma'am. A good cosmetic surgeon could make your nipples stand out for about 500 quid or so per nipple.

But I would like to stress that it is a serious symptom if a nipple inexplicably becomes inverted during adult life – and it means that you must get yourself examined by a doctor fast.

Q I am a man, and I notice that I have slight soreness and pain on passing water – plus a hint of discharge.

I have had tests and do *not* have gonorrhoea. So what could this be?

Non-specific Urethritis

Also known as NSU or non-gonococcal urethritis (NGU), this is by far the most common sexually transmitted infection in males today.

In most cases, NSU appears to be caused by the relatively 'new' organism chlamydia. Some cases may be due to other bugs, notably one called mycoplasma. The symptoms in men are:

pain on passing water

discharge from the penis.

As we'll see in a moment, those symptoms are very like these of gonorrhoea, though NSU is generally regarded as a milder infection. It can, however, have very serious complications (e.g. arthritis) in a small number of cases. Also – and very importantly – it now seems very likely that NSU in a man can make his female partner ill, or even sterile, by giving her chlamydia. Unfortunately, symptoms in *women* tend to be vague or non-existent – though there may be fever and pelvic pain.

Fortunately, treatment of NSU with one of the tetracycline group of antibiotics is usually successful. You should refrain entirely from sex until cured.

NSU

A It's important that everyone should realise that there's now a fantastically common sexually transmitted infection in this country – yet its name is not well known to the public.

It's called 'non-specific urethritis' ('NSU' for short – which must confuse certain German car manufacturers), and it's now actually more common than measles. It's usually caused by a bug called 'chlamydia'. Chlamydia isn't all that easy to test for, so many clinics simply treat men on the basis of the *symptoms* of NSU – discharge and pain passing water.

You have these symptoms, so you should now go to a VD clinic and get yourself treated immediately.

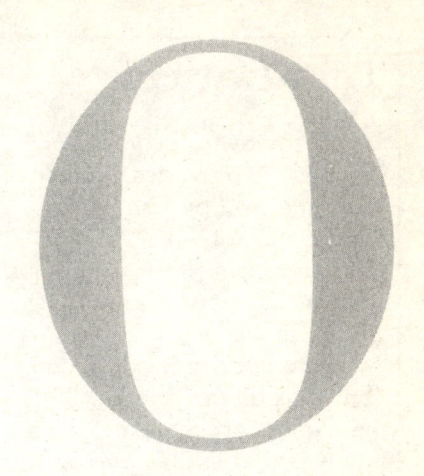

OVARIES · OVULATION

The Ovaries

Tucked away inside your pelvis, you have two ovaries. They're jolly little oval pinkish-white things, each about 3.5cm (1½") long and 2 cm (¾") across – just a bit smaller than a man's testicle, in fact.

The comparison with a man's "balls" is an apt one, because the ovaries are the exact female equivalent of the testicles, and are formed from the same tissue in the early human embryo. However, nature very sensibly tucks the ovaries away where they can't be damaged (would that she had done the same for us lads!).

Only someone with fairly long and fairly skilled fingers can feel them: they're just about palpable through the upper part of the side wall of the vagina – and some women do like having them gently stroked during love play.

Your ovaries probably contain about 100,000 eggs each, but only one egg is released each month, making a grand total of about 400 during your reproductive lifetime. Incredibly, all the rest go to waste!

Apart from releasing eggs (ovulating) the ovaries are also important sources of a woman's sex hormones – though not, curiously enough, the *only* sources. If the ovaries have to be removed, some female hormones are still manufactured in other parts of the body.

Ovulation

Ovulation means the release of an ovum (egg) from your ovary.

It happens once a month – usually about 14 days before the start of your period. A 'ripe' ovum bursts from the surface of your ovary, makes an extraordinary long jump across the enormous gap which separates the ovary from the Fallopian tube – and then belts down the tube on the off-chance of meeting an inquisitive little sperm coming up the other way!

Not too long ago, I was at a meeting which was being addressed by Robert Edwards, of Steptoe and Edwards fame.

He revealed that he has now found that ovulation nearly always takes place in the early afternoon.

Indeed, when his American patients come to Britain to

OVARIES • OVULATION

Disorders

Disorders of the ovaries are frequently difficult to diagnose, simply because of their inaccessibility.

CYSTS are very common, particularly in younger women. (Princess Anne had one removed a few years ago.) Many cysts produce no symptoms at all, but others can cause pain which can be mistaken for appendicitis.

By some weird quirk of nature, a few ovarian cysts when removed turn out to contain teeth (no kidding!).

Contrary to what many people believe, cysts of the ovary are not caused by the Pill. In fact, the Pill tends to protect you against them.

CANCER. Sadly, cancer of the ovary is quite common, and kills rather more women than the much better-known cancer of the cervix. The cause is not known, but again there is now evidence that the Pill helps to protect you against it.

Symptoms tend to be rather vague, and include persistent low abdominal pain, and bleeding after the menopause. Let me stress that the disease is rare under the age of 45.

Happily, there's a very new screening test for cancer of the ovary — it's done by ultrasound, is painless and takes only ten minutes. Unfortunately, the few ovary-screening units that offer the test are fairly swamped with patients at the moment.

---

undergo the 'test-tube baby' technique, he finds that they're ovulating at about 3pm *New York time*. But after a month or so in Britain, they start ovulating at around 3pm Greenwich Mean Time.

Edwards' announcement prompted a rash of speculation that early afternoon might be the best time to get pregnant. But don't make any arrangements for post-lunch love-making yet —

for if you think about it, the ovum usually takes a day or two to make that journey down the Fallopian tube. So provided you make love *around* the day of ovulation, there's a good chance of conceiving.

Now let's just look at what causes ovulation.

Your ovaries are about the size of small walnuts, and each of them contains the incredible figure of about 200,000 potential

OVULATION

eggs. As a rule, only one of them ripens each month (if *more* than one ripens, you may get twins).

The release of the egg is caused by a hormone signal which travels each month from your pituitary gland (at the base of your brain) to your ovaries.

Emotional stresses — or even a sudden change of work or diet — can interfere with that hormone signal, which explains why irregularity of the menstrual cycle often happens in women who've had some sort of recent upset.

You may possibly have noticed that you get a slight pain in the lower tum midway between periods; this is actually caused at the moment of ovulation by the egg being released. It's called *mittelschmertz* — which is simply German for 'middle pain'. For some women, it's a useful sign that they really are ovulating.

Women: Failure to Ovulate

For a variety of reasons, an awful lot of women do not ovulate (produce an ovum). This can be the case even though they may be having periods. So one of the first things to do in most cases of failure to conceive is to try to check whether the woman is ovulating.

A simple and cheap way of doing this is for her to take her temperature every morning over a spell of several months. If she is ovulating, her chart should register a 'kick'.

Admittedly, temperature charts can be difficult for even the most experienced doctors to interpret. In some cases, it's necessary to check whether ovulation is occurring (and — most important — *when*) by one of these methods:

hormone tests

ultrasound scan of the ovary

biopsy (sampling) of the womb lining

laparoscopy (inspecting the ovary with a telescope-like device pushed through a small cut in the abdomen).

Obviously, these methods are much more expensive (and, in most parts of the world, more difficult to obtain) than the simple temperature chart procedure.

Once a woman knows that she's ovulating — and *when* — then obviously she should make love around that day in order to conceive. But if the tests show that she's *not* ovulating, then these days there's still hope for

OVULATION

P

her.

Failure to ovulate can very often be successfully treated with the famous 'fertility drugs' – which stimulate the ovary to produce eggs. Most of these drugs mimic the action of the natural hormones which are produced by a woman's pituitary gland, which should make her ovary produce an ovum each month.

Unfortunately, as you probably know from the newspapers, use of certain fertility drugs does often over-stimulate the ovaries, so that they produce *too many* eggs. The result is a multiple pregnancy; indeed in a few cases, the fertility drugs have had the startling effect of giving the woman up to eight babies.

I'm afraid that the survival rate of the babies in these extreme cases of multiple pregnancy is low.

Obviously, infertility specialists try to control the dose of fertility drug very carefully so that if possible only one, two or at most three babies are produced at a single pregnancy.

Usually (though not invariably), a woman who has been desperately trying for a baby over a period of many years is usually only too delighted if she ends up with twins or even triplets!

PELVIC FLOOR MUSCLES • PENIS

Q I am in my mid-50s, and last year had a pelvic floor repair operation. Prior to the operation, the surgeon did warn me that intercourse might be difficult.

It's not difficult — it's *impossible*, because I am now so tight! Will things improve with time, or would you advise me to get my husband one of those inflatable dolls?

A Well, congratulations on your sense of humour, ma'am! A well-performed pelvic repair op usually makes intercourse better — not worse; you should go back to the surgeon, or get a second opinion. A 're-fashioning' operation might be necessary. But it's possible you could be helped by either female hormone cream or vaginal relaxation exercises — or possibly through the use of graduated dilators which stretch the tissues. Good luck.

Q I am an 18-year-old male and I am worried because my penis is bent to one side when it is erect. I could not see my doctor about this.

A Well, I'm afraid you're going

The Pelvic Floor Muscles

Lots of people don't really understand what the pelvic floor muscles are. Indeed, recently I had a slightly surreal conversation with an otherwise highly-informed woman who thought that pelvic floor exercises were so called because you had to do them on the floor!

The pelvic floor is a cleverly interwoven basket of muscle which forms a network that supports the organs in the pelvis — including the womb, ovaries and bladder. You can get a rough idea of the size and shape of the muscles of the pelvic floor simply by holding your two hands palms upwards in front of you. Then slide the two hands together, so that the fingers interlock. The resulting shallow basin is quite like the pelvic floor. Imagine that it's supporting your pelvic organs and that there are two apertures in the basin, through which pass the vagina and the rectum.

It's very important for all women to know about this pelvic floor musculature because in so many ladies, childbirth leads to serious *weakening* of these muscles — with unfortunate consequ-

PELVIC FLOOR MUSCLES

ences for love-life and health. Repeated childbirth and *difficult* and *prolonged* labours are particularly likely to do this. As far as her sex life is concerned, a woman is likely to find that her vagina seems to have become slack and loose.

Furthermore, severe weakness of these muscles can lead to *prolapse* (descent of the womb); much more frequently, it simply causes problems with urination and the woman may find that she has embarrassing incontinence, especially when she coughs or laughs.

Gross weakness of the pelvic floor muscles can usually be put right, with one of a variety of surgical repair operations. Obviously, it's much better to avoid surgery altogether, and this can be done by means of pelvic floor exercises.

Every woman should do these exercises daily for several months after the birth of a child. Any woman who feels that her vagina is a little too loose can do these exercises – they are quite good fun, and they may prevent the need for a vaginal repair operation later on in life. The exercises develop the muscles just where they surround the vagina, and where they grip the penis during intercourse.

Indeed, the exercises can and should be done during intercourse: this is enjoyable, and your partner will find it pleasant too. Once these muscles are strengthened, you'll discover that doing the exercises creates an agreeable sort of 'milking' sensation in his male organ. But it's no good just doing the exercises during love-making. As with any other 'muscle building' exercises, *you need to do them for about 20 minutes twice a day – over at least six months*.

You can do the two exercises while you're at work, or pushing a pram, or sitting in the bath – no one will know you're doing them. Here they are:

Exercise one: make a real effort to tighten up the *front* part of your pelvic muscles, by 'tightening up' as if you were trying to stop yourself passing water. Hold the contraction for 10 seconds, then release for 10 seconds. Continue for 10 minutes.

Exercise two: make a similar effort to contract the back part of your pelvic floor muscles by 'tightening up' as if to hold back a bowel movement. Again, maintain the contraction for 10 seconds, then relax for 10 seconds – repeat for 10 minutes.

PENIS

The Penis

Now to the organ which so many people get concerned about: the penis.

It's surprising that this particular organ generates such a lot of emotion, embarrassment and even outrage. For after all, it's a somewhat unimpressive little structure, comparing rather unfavourably in dimensions with a decent-sized *andouillette*.

However, one has to face the fact that many men and women do have hang-ups about the penis. In the case of men, vast numbers have an extraordinary obsession about penis size – and are firmly convinced that their own is too small. In the case of women, a surprising number of females feel frightened or disgusted by the idea of a close encounter with a male organ.

You may be surprised to hear it, but some wives are so emotional about this matter that they cannot bring themselves to touch their husbands' penises.

Perhaps life would be easier if everybody understood a few of the basic facts about this organ. The penis is the male equivalent of a woman's clitoris. It's equipped with a great many 'pleasure receptors' which, when stimulated, produce very agreeable sensations in the man's brain.

The average penis in its non-erect state is quite a bit smaller than most people imagine. In general, it measures between 8.5cm (just over 3ins) and 10.5cm (just over 4ins) – but it varies a lot, depending on the weather.

Masters and Johnson have discovered a curious fact of which few men are aware. Though penises vary quite a bit in size in the non-erect state, they are to have to – because no one else is going to straighten this out for you.

In fact, your doc will probably send you to a specialist called a urologist, who will be able to tell you whether there is anything wrong, or whether this is just a slight variation from normal.

Urologists see a lot of blokes who are worried because their penises develop a bend when they become erect. Since a specialist can hardly examine a man during an erection, some urologists actually ask men to bring in a Polaroid photo of the erect penis – so that they can assess the degree of bend.

Please don't worry too much about this – but you definitely do need a medical opinion.

PERIOD PAINS

nearly all about the same size when they are erect. So though many males feel inadequate about the size of their penis, this is all quite unnecessary — especially as most women are not remotely interested.

The penis is a very simple structure in comparison with the female genital organs. It consists of three 'cylinders' of tissue, which are capable of filling with blood (thus causing an erection.

On the end of these three cylinders is the cone-shaped glans, which is the most sexually sensitive part.

The only other thing to say about the penis is that contrary to what so many women (and men) imagine, it's actually a pretty clean structure. Provided a man washes regularly under his foreskin (if uncircumcised) there should be nothing 'dirty' about it.

Q What's the best treatment for period pain?

A It's usual to start with aspirin or paracetamol, or one of the vast number of formulations based on them.

But, if that doesn't work, some

Period Problems

The menses, or periods, begin at about the age of 12 on average, though many girls experience the first menstruation as early as 10 or as late as 16. (If the periods start before 10, or if they haven't started by the 17th birthday, always check with the doctor.) Menstruation continues until the change of life, which means that the average woman will have something like 400 periods.

One still finds patients who think that the female cycle is somehow linked to the calendar (or even to the Moon!), and who therefore expect their periods to arrive on the same day of every calendar month. In fact, the menstrual cycle is usually considerably less than a full month in length — 26 days from start to start being about the average. Quite a lot of women have cycles as short as 16 days, or as long as 40 days, and some have periods only once every few months or so.

Irregular and Heavy Periods

It really doesn't matter all that much how long the menstrual cycle is. (There is nothing especially 'right' about a 26-day or

PERIOD PAINS

28-day cycle, as a lot of people think.) All that is important is that the periods should be reasonably regular, and that blood loss should not be excessive.

If the periods are irregular, you should always consult a doctor. Nobody need expect their period to come with split-second timing each cycle, but a woman ought to be able to forecast the arrival of her menses to within about two or three days.

Bleeding between the periods or bleeding after intercourse are possible *danger signs* and must not be ignored. See your doctor, who will probably perform an examination and, if necessary, refer you to a gynaecologist.

Heavy periods are not only a nuisance but are liable to cause excessive loss of iron, with resultant anaemia. It is largely because women have periods that they're so much more liable to anaemia than men are.

It's hard to say what constitutes heavy loss in any individual case, but if you are getting 'flooding' (*i.e.* if tampons and towels don't seem to be coping with the flow very well), or if regular bleeding goes on for more than six days each month, or if you are getting unusually pale or unusually tired and breathless, then it's definitely

doctors believe in prescribing an anti-spasmodic called Buscopan. A successful trend in recent years has been to try anti-rheumatic drugs such as Ponstan and Naprosyn.

However, by far the most successful abolisher of period pain in Britain is the Pill. Most younger women who suffer from dysmen find that a correctly chosen brand of the Pill wipes it out.

Some people are not very keen on taking the Pill, and ask for other hormones instead. But the truth is that these are usually Pill-type hormones under another name – and probably have similar side-effects.

Commonsense measures include a hot water bottle on the tummy or the back – and gentle massage of the same areas.

A feminist group recently raised a few eyebrows by suggesting that rubbing one's own clitoris would help. Acupuncture is also useful, but rather less fun.

Q How I wish I could just bring on my period each month on exactly the day when *I* want it!

It would be nice just to 'flush

PERIOD PAINS

best to check with your doctor. He will examine you, and probably do a simple blood test to find out if your body's iron stores have been depleted by excessive menstrual bleeding. If so, it shouldn't be too difficult to put things right. The Pill and similar hormone preparations can, of course, have side-effects – but they are very, very effective in treating heavy, prolonged and irregular periods.

Painful Periods

Pain with periods can be very troublesome indeed. In the past, it was something of a fashion for (male!) doctors to say that much of the distress was purely psychological, and that if the girl would only pull herself together all would be well. This was (literally) bloody silly.

Period pain is often absent when the menses first start, but may begin a few months later. The reason for this is that in the early menstrual cycles, there is often no ovulation (see below), and in many patients ovulation seems to be necessary for menstrual pain to occur.

This is why taking the Pill is often a cure for painful periods, since it suppresses ovulation. That provides an effective

everything away' every four weeks, and not have to worry endlessly about contraception.

Why haven't you doctors come up with anything convenient like that?

A Sorry! In fact, there is a French tablet which will do more or less what you say. It's called RU468.

It does give women the power to control their own fertility – and to bring on a period when they want one. But, unfortunately, as with every other drug, there are side-effects. *And because the tablet is regarded by many people as an abortifacient, there's bound to be a heck of an ethical row about releasing it in Britain.*

Pro-life MPs have recently started asking questions about the new drug – and they appear to have obtained assurances from the manufacturers that RU468 WON'T be sold over the counter to British women. It also seems likely that a British woman who wants to use it will have to get two doctors to sign an Abortion Act form first.

If this is true, my personal forecast is that feminists will try to smuggle it in from France.

PERIODS

method of treatment, but in younger girls with only relatively mild period symptoms, it's often best to begin treatment with simple analgesic drugs. A large number of preparations are now available for the relief of period pain, and the doctor will often try quite a variety before he finds a suitable one. If pain is bad, there should be no hesitation about taking the day off school or work and retiring to bed. A hot water bottle clasped to the tummy will often provide a lot of relief. Anti-inflammatory drugs like Ponstan may be helpful.

Ovulation and Periods

You need to understand the relationship of ovulation (the release of an egg from the ovary) to the menses, since ovulation is the time at which conception occurs.

Most of the time, in most women, ovulation happens a little before the half-way point of the menstrual cycle. For a woman whose periods are 26 days apart, therefore, the likeliest time for conception is about 11 to 13 days after the start of a period.

Ovulation varies a lot, however, and there is no way of being *sure*. A slight backache is sometimes a clue to the fact that it is taking place. Some patients take their temperature every morning before getting up and record the results on a chart. A little 'kick' upwards on the graph (preceded by a slight dip) very often occurs on the day of ovulation.

It is also possible to buy 'conception-day indicators', simple calculating devices into which one feeds data concerning the length of recent menstrual cycles. As a way of reckoning the conception day they are not as effective as the temperature chart method.

The time at which conception is *least* likely is just before and during the menses. Some people call this time the 'safe period', but this is a bit misleading; there are hundreds of thousands of children in the world who owe their existence to the fact that their parents believed in the 'safe period'! All that can be said is that it is probably safer than any other time of the cycle. Many Catholic women (and others) swear by the 'Billings' version of the 'safe period', in which you plot the nature of your vaginal secretions on a daily chart.

THE PILL

Q Is it true that the Pill gives you cancer of the liver? I have been on it for three years, and have always been very careful to have regular check-ups. My doctor assured me that I was on a 'low-dose' brand which could not possibly cause side-effects.

But last week I read a newspaper report which said that doctors had found that it caused liver cancer.

I made an appointment to see my doctor and asked him if I should have tests for liver cancer, but he just laughed at me.

A Oh, dear – a rather unfortunate response, I fear. But, in fact, nobody who is taking the Pill needs to have tests for liver cancer.

However, papers in the *British Medical Journal* have suggested a possible (but very, very minute) risk of liver cancer from long-term use of the Pill. Naturally, this has caused some newspaper headlines.

Though this complication is very rare, any woman who gets persistent tummy pain or jaundice while on the Pill should see her doc urgently.

However, one final point: despite what your doc says, there's no such thing as a Pill which 'could not possibly cause side-effects.'

Q I get very depressed on the Pill. Have you any suggestions?

A Well, if you definitely feel that the depression is due to the Pill, then either come off it or switch to a totally different brand.

Alternatively, some women who become depressed on the Pill do feel they can combat it by taking pyridoxine (vitamin B_6). Your doctor may be willing to prescribe this, or else you can buy it without prescription at the chemist's.

But although there's a lot to be said in favour of the Pill, it's crazy to keep on taking it if you get depression or other severe side-effects.

Q My girlfriend has decided that she shouldn't go on the Pill. Would it be safe if we made love unprotected within ten days of her period starting?

A No – if you do this, she will in all probability get pregnant. If you want to use the 'rhythm method', then go and get some medical advice about how to use it properly. (And I warn you – it isn't easy.)

THE PILL

The Pill

The Pill remains fantastically popular in most western countries. For instance, in Britain there was a time quite recently when a startling *one in three* of all women of child-bearing age was taking it!

But although the Pill has been in widespread use for many years (it was invented in 1956), there are still worries about it – and new facts are constantly coming to light about it. So it's better not to go on it unless you've fully discussed any doubts you may have with your doctor or clinic.

Having said that, I have to add that the Pill is probably the most outstandingly successful contraceptive of all time. Taken properly – which means for 21 days out of every 28 – it will give you virtually 100% protection against pregnancy.

It does this because it contains two female-type hormones (an oestrogen and a progestogen). These affect the pituitary gland – at the base of the brain – so that it no longer sends out signals telling your ovaries to ovulate.

Side-effects

Most women who go on the Pill get no side-effects. But during the first few packs a substantial number do experience headache, nausea, breast tenderness, weight gain or bleeding between periods.

Serious side-effects are rare. But cases of thrombosis (clots) can be *fatal*. The danger of this happening is much greater in smokers, in more mature (35-plus) women, and in those with certain other risk factors. *Heavy smokers should never take the Pill*. Even moderate smokers should try to give up this dangerous habit.

The relation of the Pill to cancer is very complex. At the time of writing, it *appears* (and I stress the word *appears*) that the Pill probably helps protect you against two types of cancer – of the ovary and the womb lining – but *may* increase the risk of other types, including cancer of the cervix and (in younger women) of the breast.

Make sure you discuss any worrying reports with your doctor or clinic – and take advantage of regular smear tests for cancer of the cervix which all Pill-prescribing doctors or clinics can arrange.

Finally, after all these warn-

THE PILL

ings, do bear in mind that the Pill does have certain very *good* effects. In particular, a well-chosen brand should make your periods painless, shorter and lighter.

The mini-Pill

The mini-Pill is used mainly by women who no longer wish to take the Pill (e.g. the over-35s) and by breast-feeding mothers (this is because, unlike the ordinary Pill, it doesn't suppress milk production).

It is not a low-dose version of the ordinary Pill, but is a quite different thing, containing only one hormone (a progestogen) instead of two.

At the moment, it does appear to be much 'milder' than the ordinary Pill, and complaints of side-effects are much lower. Disruption of the periods is the chief possible side-effect: they may become too far apart, or irritatingly frequent!

The mini-Pill seems to work *mainly* by thickening the secretions in the cervix, making it difficult for sperm to get through. You must — repeat *must* — take it *every single day at about the same time, without any breaks at all.*

It's at maximum effectiveness about 6 to 8 hours after you take it. So if you usually make love in the late evening, you'll get the best protection by taking your mini-Pill each day at around 4 pm.

One word of warning: although the mini-Pill's reputation is as a very mild contraceptive, it *is* nonetheless a hormone. This means that its long-term effects will not be known for a long time to come. If in doubt, discuss any anxieties you may have with your doctor or clinic.

The Vaginal Pill

In the mid-1980s, world-wide interest was aroused by the announcement that a Brazilian researcher, Professor Coutinho, was giving the Pill by the vaginal route. (It can easily be absorbed by the vaginal tissues.)

This may seem a bit strange, but the basic idea is, in theory, not a bad one. Taking the Pill in this way does prevent one of itscommon side-effects, namely nausea.

THE PILL

I had the entertaining experience of being at the meeting where Professor Coutinho first presented his findings at the Royal College of Obstetricians and Gynaecologists in London, at which he suggested that a major British trial of his vaginal Pill should now take place.

A questioner from the floor leapt up and declared that this method of adminstering the Pill would *not* be acceptable to British women. She added that if anyone set up a trial in the UK, there would be a high rate of drop-out.

'*Drop-out?*' thundered Professor Coutinho, misunderstanding completely. 'Certainly not — my Pills do not drop out!'

The New French Monthly Pill

In 1985, the world was startled by reports from France of a new once-a-month pill, which a woman could simply use every 28 days to 'clear out' he womb. It was alleged to be 100% effective. Quite understandably, this idea aroused a lot of indignation among people who regarded the new French invention as a licence to carry out do-it-yourself abortion — which would make it unacceptable to a very large number of women. Indeed, in late 1988 'pro-life' pressure forced the manufacturers to stop making it. Then the French Government ordered them to carry on!

I have talked to Professor Baulieu, the French inventor of this new pill — which at the moment is usually known as RU468. He recently told me that while he has high hopes for his invention, it's probably only about 95% effective at the moment, and it has to be used in combination with strong drugs called prostaglandins.

This makes do-it-yourself administration rather more difficult. Also, both RU468 and the prostaglandins are powerful drugs; all past experience suggests to me that there could be long-term side-effects.

Q I want to go on the Pill, and would like to know what is the safest, please.

A Unfortunately, it's still impossible to say which of the 25 or so brands of the Pill is the safest.

THE PILL

It is known that the old 'high-dose' brands of Pill were more dangerous from the point of view of causing thrombosis. But after I complained about them in this column some years ago, a question was asked in the House of Commons. Soon afterwards, they were all taken off the market.

Today, most Pills are 'low dose', though a few are 'medium dose' (50 microgrammes).

Most GPs and Family Planning Clinics tend to prescribe the low-dose pills for the majority of women.

Q I am on the Pill and I'm going abroad soon. Will I be able to get the same Pill in other countries?

A Probably not, but there are equivalent brands. For details of brand names, contact the International Planned Parenthood Federation on 01-486 0741.

Q I keep forgetting to take my Pill. What should I do in order to avoid getting pregnant?

A If you keep forgetting to take it, then maybe you should be on some other form of contraception. But obviously, everyone forgets their Pill occasionally.

The latest FPA advice on how to cope with this common situation is as follows:

If you're more than 12 hours late taking your Pill, you could be at risk of pregnancy. You should take *extra* precautions (like using a condom – or not having sex) for the next seven days.

If you missed the Pill during *the last week* of your packet, then it's best not to have a break between that pack and the next one.

Q Is it really true that the Pill can be taken vaginally?

A Yes, it is true – and taking it by this rather bizarre route does mean that you avoid one of the very common side-effects of the Pill – namely nausea.

But the danger is that you wouldn't be able to get the Pill far enough up; there's also a risk that its coating might not dissolve quickly enough for the contraceptive to be effective.

And your chap might be unfortunate enough to absorb a dose of it when he made love to you! So please, I warn you, don't attempt to try this lark without medical supervision.

THE PILL

Q I will soon be 35, and therefore unable to take the Pill any longer. I don't want to use one of those coil things, and my husband dislikes any kind of rubbery contraception. Can you suggest anything?

A Well, vast numbers of women are encountering this problem at the moment – now that doctors are tending to take many women off the Pill at about 35. But the No Pill After 35 rule certainly isn't an absolute one. The risk of being killed by the Pill doesn't suddenly shoot upwards on your 35th birthday; in reality, it seems to increase very slightly throughout your 30s and 40s. So some women do stay on the Pill for a little while after they're 35. But when the time comes to *stop* taking the Pill, the solution for many women these days is the mini-Pill. This is not – repeat *not* – a low-dose version of the ordinary Pill; it's a quite different thing. Basically, it's a tablet that contains just one hormone, instead of the two hormones in the ordinary Pill. It's free of oestrogen – a fact which appears to make it less risky. Indeed, at the time of writing (touch wood) no one has ever had a fatal thrombosis caused by the mini-Pill. So talk to your doctor or clinic about the possibility of switching to the mini-Pill.

Because so many people are muddled about just which brands are mini-Pills and which *aren't*, I'm going to list the available ones here. They are: Femulen; Micronor; Microval; Neogest; Norgeston; and Noriday.

Q Whenever I go and see my doctor to get a prescription for the Pill, she seems to be obsessed with how much I smoke. Is there some connection between smoking and the Pill?

A Yes – I'm constantly amazed at how few people realise this. Smoking is not only dangerous in itself, but it also increases the risks of the Pill considerably. One major British study suggests that if a Pill-taker starts smoking, she may become eight times as likely to die of a heart attack or stroke.

So if you want to go on taking the Pill, the best thing is to give up the dreaded weed altogether. Smoking is a mind-bogglingly stupid habit – and especially so for somebody on the Pill.

Q A year ago I was forced to stop taking the Pill because my blood pressure had risen considerably. Since then, my boyfriend

THE PILL

and I *have not* enjoyed having to use the diaphragm.

Is there any type of Pill which is freer of side-effects?

A Well, it'd certainly be worth asking your doctor to tell you about the 'mini-Pill'.

That's the one-hormone only Pill which you have to take every single day, but which is generally milder than the ordinary Pill.

I can't guarantee that it'd suit you, but it's worth considering.

Q I am thinking of going on the Pill, since most of my girl friends seem to be on it. But does it cause cancer?

A At the time of writing, there isn't as much worry about the relationship between the Pill and cancer as there was during the last 'Pill scare'. Also, it has become clear that the Pill almost certainly protects women to some extent against two particular types of cancer.

But the Pill certainly hasn't got a clean bill of health, and I have to admit that there are still serious question marks over the link with breast and cervix cancer.

This is a bit worrying, since three million British women still take the Pill and are theoretically at risk (it remains the most popular method in the UK, in fact).

So if you do choose the Pill, you should take even more care than other women to do two things: (a) check your breasts regularly for lumps; (b) have regular smears done.

But remember, this should be your own decision. Clearly you shouldn't go on the Pill just because your friends are on it.

Q Is it true that as I am a contact lens wearer, I must not take the Pill?

A Nope. This is a common myth, but there's no reason why contact-lens wearers shouldn't take the Pill.

However, some contact users do find difficulties with their lenses when they first start the Pill. This is probably because of increased fluid retention in the eyeball, but it's not usually much of a problem.

Q I'm going on the Pill. How often should I have check-ups?

A Opinions differ, but most

PINWORMS • PMT

authorities say that you should be seen by a doc or nurse every six months — particularly to discuss 'risk factors' like smoking and high blood pressure.

Frequency of internal examinations and breast checks depends a lot on what facilities are available in your area. At many hard-pressed NHS clinics 'internals' tend to be done about every three years. Breast checks may be omitted altogether, I'm afraid, so it's best to make sure that you know how to do your own check-up each month.

Q I have recently picked up what appear to be white worms round my bottom. They make me itch at night, and are very uncomfortable. I am too embarrassed to go to my doctor, so could you please tell me what to do to get rid of them?

A These are almost certainly threadworms (pinworms), which are very common. If you have any children, you may have picked up the worms from them.

They live in the lower part of the bowel, and come out of the bottom at night to lay their eggs on the skin — which is why the itching is always nocturnal.

There's been recent discussion in medical journals about how the threadworms KNOW that it's night-time? (After all, it's always dark up your bottom.)

Anyway, what happens next is that you scratch your underneath parts — and get eggs trapped under your fingernails.

If you're not careful, it's then easy to transfer the eggs to someone else's mouth (eg: on food) — or to re-infect yourself via your own mouth.

I think you should see your doc to get the diagnosis confirmed — especially as the odds are that the whole family will need treating (usually with a drug called piperazine).

Q I have very bad PMT which is driving my husband up the wall. My doctor has been treating me for several years with Cyclogest suppositoires. Is there anything else?

A Yup. Cyclogest *suppositoires* are OK, but they're not everybody's cup of tea, so to speak.

Other treatments for PMT include the hormone dydrogesterone, Vitamin B_6, diuretics ('water pills'), and Efamol capsules. I suggest you talk these possibilities over with your doc.

There's also an advisory service for people with pre-menstrual ten-

PREGNANCY • POST-NATAL CHECK

sion, which stresses the alleged nutritional basis of the problem. They have produced a book 'Beat PMT Through Diet' — £5.99 Ebury Press, but I don't know of any very convincing evidence that it will help you.

Q I went to my doctor recently for a post-natal check, and was surprised that he did not examine me internally.

A That's very odd indeed. I take it that he wasn't one of these SAS-type doctors — trained to get in and out without anyone noticing.

More seriously, you do need an internal examination after you've had a baby, just to check that everything's back to normal. (You may also be due for a smear.)

If it's awkward to return to this doc and demand an internal, then

---

Pregnancy and Sex

It's quite common for women suddenly to lose interest in sex either during pregnancy or immediately after it.

This reaction may be partly due to hormone changes. It can also be linked to the stress and tiredness which affect so many women during pregnancy, childbirth, and the months afterwards.

There may also be a psychological element. A number of women do have a feeling deep down that sex is all right for young women — but that once you become a mother (or a mother-to-be) then you really shouldn't enjoy it any more!

In many cases, this loss of interest cures itself — especially if the couple talk about it together and the man adopts a sensible and sympathetic attitude.

Incidentally, the great weight of medical opinion nowadays is that there is no reason at all why you shouldn't make love during pregnancy. Provided there are no abnormalities in the course of the pregnancy (e.g. bleeding) there seems to be no harm in making love as late as you like. A recent study in the *New England Journal of Medicine* seems to indicate that babies of couples who made love late in pregnancy are just as healthy as those of couples who didn't.

However, when you get very big, sex in the orthodox positions can be uncomfortable. You may prefer to restrict yourselves to love-play when pregnancy is far advanced.

PROLAPSE • PROSTATE

I suggest you make an appointment with your local Well-Woman or Family Planning Clinic (I've checked, and there's one not far from you). If you explain the situation, they'll most likely be pleased to oblige.

Q I am horrified to find that my doctor has just diagnosed a prolapse. Is it due to having too much sex?

A A prolapse is a general sort of collapsing downwards of your internal sex organs, caused by weakness of the supporting tissues.

It's *not* caused by sex – but by childbirth (and particularly *repeated* childbirth).

It is slightly less common than it used to be, mainly because women are having smaller families these days. Exercises may help in mild cases – such as the excellent ones provided by the self-help groups which have recently sprung up in women's gym classes.

But if your case is more severe, I'm afraid you'll need a 'tightening up' operation, to take in a few 'tucks' and try to restore you to your former state of beauty.

Q I read your recent article about the prostate gland. I am a man who has had this operation, and I would like to say that what no one ever tells you is that after it has been done, the ejaculatory function is lost. The feeling at

Prostate Gland

This is a gland about the size of a large chestnut which lies at the neck of the male bladder. There is no exactly corresponding structure in women, though recent research suggests that the G-spot in women is a very similar organ. The prostate gland produces a liquid that forms part of the seminal fluid.

The urinary passage goes right through the prostate, and the unfortunate consequence of this is that enlargement of the gland will block the flow of urine from the bladder, either completely or partially.

The cause of the enlargement of the prostate is not known, but, like greying of the hair, and stiffness of the joints, it's probably just another consequence of ageing. It doesn't seem to affect sexual function.

The patient with an enlarged prostate usually notices that he has some difficulty in producing a good stream of urine, and that

PROSTATE

orgasm is still there, but there is no ejaculation.

AWell, you're quite right, sir. If the prostate gland is removed (or if a substantial amount is 'nibbled away' with a surgical instrument) you do not ejaculate. This is disappointing and irritating to quite a few men.

It's a pity that the surgeon didn't explain this to you beforehand – though I think that most men would have gone ahead with the op anyway.

sometimes it may be very difficult to 'get started', particularly when the bladder is full. Most patients are obliged to get up once or twice at night to pass water.

There is also a risk of *acute retention* developing; in this condition, no urine can get out of the bladder at all and prompt treatment is necessary.

Treatment of an Enlarged Prostate

GENERAL. Many mild cases of prostatic enlargement can be kept in check by simple means. If you have a moderately enlarged prostate, you should avoid drinking large quantities of fluid, particularly alcohol, tea and coffee, all of which tend to increase the flow of urine. (These drinks are quite all right in moderation, however.)

Make sure you empty your bladder regularly – say, every one to two hours, and especially before setting off on long journeys. The worst possible thing to do, for instance, would be to have several pints of beer before a long, unbroken car ride home on a cold night – this would be inviting an attack of acute retention.

Another important point to remember is that prostate sufferers are particularly liable to inflammation of the bladder or cystitis and, in fact, any kind of urinary infection. So, if you get pain and discomfort on passing water, see your doctor as soon as possible, so that he can send a carefully collected specimen of urine to the lab for culture.

SURGICAL. When prostate trouble gets too bad, surgery is essential. About one prostate patient in four eventually needs an operation. It's now often possible to carry out what's called a TUR (or transurethral resection), which simply involves pushing a slim telescope with a cutting device up the urinary passage, and nibbling away bits of the prostate so as to make the passage wider. But the surgeon may operate to remove the *whole* prostate gland.

This procedure (prostatectomy, as it's called) at one time used to be very dangerous, and very distressing for the patient. Nowadays, it's a straightforward and safe business, though the few days after the operation are not usually much fun.

Most patients do very well, however, and are out of hospital within about two weeks. A month or so of convalescence will be required. Urinary control should usually be regained shortly after the operation.

With luck there will be only partial interference with sexual function, and some men, because of improved general good health, actually enjoy happier marital relations after the operation. Seminal fluid will no longer be produced at orgasm, which means that the man will probably be unable to have further children. Since most patients are at least in their late fifties, and have long completed their fami-

Pruritus

Pruritus literally means itching, but the word is often used to mean itching of either the vaginal opening (*pruritus vulvae*) or of the back passage (*pruritus ani*).

Vulval and Vaginal Pruritus

Itching of the vulva and vagina is a trying and embarrassing symptom for many women. There are various possible causes. It may be necessary to examine the urine for sugar (which might indicate diabetes). Bacteriological swabs from the vagina should usually be sent to the lab, particularly if there is a discharge present, as is often the case. Frequently, examination of these swabs will reveal the presence of thrush (also known as Monilia or Candida) or of another organism called *Trichomonas vaginalis*, sometimes confusingly known as TV.

Other causes of irritation in this area include fungus infections, and other skin inflammations, as well as allergy to vaginal deodorants, contraceptive foams, soaps and bubble baths.

Anal Pruritus

Irritation of the back passage is

PUBIC HAIR

lies, this is not usually of any consequence.

Cancer of the Prostate

When a patient who has symptoms of prostate trouble seeks medical advice, the doctor should always do a rectal examination, since this enables him to feel the size, shape and texture of the gland with his finger. If the gland feels craggy and hard, cancer may be present, but I must stress that cancer is *rare* compared with ordinary benign enlargement of the gland.

Cure of prostatic cancer can be achieved by complete removal of the gland. Some patients are treated with hormones.

Some doctors, especially in the US, feel that all males over the age of 50 should have a yearly rectal examination to detect both benign and malignant disease of the prostate, as well as disorders of the rectum itself. Lives could probably be saved by this sort of universal screening, but the costs would be huge.

---

a very widespread problem, especially in men. A lot of doctors think that psychological factors play a part in at least some cases, but they could be wrong! Physical factors include inflamed piles and anal eczema, which is very common and responds well to steroid ointments.

Threadworms and fungus infections can produce intense pruritus, and the symptoms can also follow the taking of antibiotics by mouth. Over-vigorous wiping of the anal region after defaecation can also lead to irritation, as can sitting for far too long in hot baths.

Q My lack of hair in the pubic area has made my life a misery.

Why? Because my second-ever lover spread the word around our town that I was hairless in this region, and it made me a 'local joke'.

Since then, I have never been able to go out with anyone, and I have become very lonely and depressed.

A I'm so sorry to hear about this. It's appalling that your former lover treated you like this.

If you really have practically no hair around the 'pubes', then you may be suffering from a hormone

PUBIC HAIR

deficiency, which might be put right.

I can't guarantee this – but I do think that you should ask your doc if she'll refer you to an endocrinologist (that's a gland specialist) to see if hormone therapy would help.

If not – well, bear in mind that many men actually LIKE a girl to have 'bare pubes' and enthusiastically beg their partners to shave it all off! So have courage – I'm sure all will be well.

Q Would it be all right to shampoo my pubic hair? I always feel that mine is rather thick and 'crinkly', and that this will put men off.

A I'm sure it won't – after all, pubic hair is supposed to be deep and crisp and even (as they say).

But there's no reason at all why you shouldn't shampoo your 'pubes' with ordinary hair shampoo – and put conditioner on as well if you like!

In fact, I'm surprised that some enterprising shampoo manufacturer hasn't already come up with a special brand for this area.

Stop Press: As this book went to press, I learned that pubic shampoos have just reached the shops.

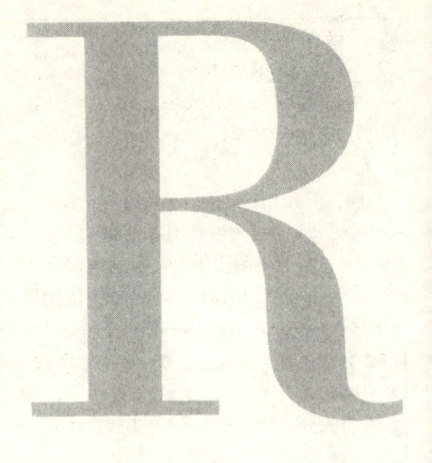

RHYTHM METHOD

Q Is it true that there's a new, 100% reliable version of the 'rhythm method?'

A Nope. But large companies have made significant advances towards developing a 'home test', which would enable a woman to pinpoint her own ovulation day.

I reckon it'll be at least several years before they get the bugs ironed out. But when they do, it'll be a great boost for the 'rhythm method' – not to mention the Catholic Church.

Rhythm – and Other 'Natural' Methods

'Natural' methods are the only ones which are at the moment acceptable to the Catholic Church. It's true that in recent years there has also been more interest in them among non-Catholic couples – partly as a result of understandable worries about the Pill and other hormonal contraceptives.

However, the proportion of couples outside Catholic countries who use natural methods is still very low indeed – probably less than 1%. To be frank, I am not surprised, because the failure rate of these methods is very high, except among those who are extremely well motivated.

Natural methods fall into two groups: rhythm, and lactation.

Rhythm Methods

Rhythm or the 'safe period' techniques depend on avoiding love-making at the time when the woman is most likely to be fertile. This tends to be in the 'middle' of the menstrual month – in other words, roughly halfway between periods.

Unfortunately, however, women *can* ovulate at almost any time of the month, so if you want to use the rhythm method, it is best to employ some method that will help you to identify the 'danger days' with reasonable accuracy.

Quite soon now, science will find a cheap and convenient way in which any woman can pinpoint her day of ovulation. But until then the best ways of estimating your safe and 'danger' periods are:

the temperature chart method

the Billings method.

The *temperature chart method* relies on taking your temperature every morning, and plotting it

255

RHYTHM METHOD

with great accuracy on a specially designed chart.

The *Billings method* was invented by two Australian doctors, John and Evelyn Billings, and involves plotting the nature of your vaginal secretions on a chart. The idea is that, on certain days of the cycle, when the vaginal secretion is clear, slippery and 'stretchy', fertilization is very likely, and sex should therefore be avoided.

Learning to identify the nature of your secretions correctly takes time, patience, intelligence and commitment. It also requires careful *training* by someone who knows what they're doing. So do not attempt the Billings technique by yourselves. If you decide to try it, both of you should attend one of the special 'Billings Clinics', which (in the UK) are often run in co-operation with Catholic Marriage Advisory Councils.

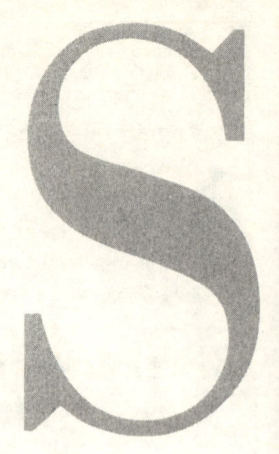

Salpingitis

This is inflammation of the Fallopian tubes, which run from the ovaries to the womb. It is caused by infection with germs, and may be either acute or chronic (*i.e.* long-lasting).

Acute Salpingitis

This is a common cause of acute abdominal pain. The chief symptoms are pain in the lower abdomen (either right-sided or left-sided, depending on which tube is involved) and fever, with a temperature of perhaps 102°F (38.9°C). There will often have been a vaginal discharge and some menstrual irregularity in the preceding few weeks.

The patient is usually admitted to hospital. With the correct antibiotic treatment, the outlook is good and most people are well on the road to recovery within a couple of weeks.
See also: CHLAMYDIA.

Chronic Salpingitis

This is a long-standing inflammation, which may follow infection of the tubes during childbirth or abortion (miscarriage). It may sometimes be due to gonorrhoea, especially where the original infection produced no symptoms. Another common cause is Chlamydia.

The features of this condition are variable but include intermittent pain low in the abdomen, vaginal discharge, irregular and painful periods, and sterility.

The skilled care of a gynaecologist is essential. Surgery is sometimes helpful, but prolonged medical treatment may be required.

The Shot

In the west, a very small number of women use the Shot (also known as the 'Jab'), though it has been employed on a wide scale in Third World countries. It has long been fully legalized in Britain, though in America the FDA have reiterated their objections to it over many years, because of doubts about possible long-term side-effects.

It's an injection that prevents you from getting pregnant, and gives virtually 100% protection. The injection is a hormone of the progestogen type (that is, like

THE SHOT

one of the two hormones in the Pill). By far the most common brand worldwide is Depo-Provera (also known as medroxyprogesterone acetate). A less widely used brand is Noristerat (norethisterone oenanthate).

Women's groups in many countries have got very indignant about Depo-Provera, and have waged highly successful campaigns against its use. I must say that I have to agree with two of their objections.

Firstly, the drug has all too often been given to women 'routinely' without any mention of possible side-effects. (Many women in Britain were at one time given it post-natally without ever realizing that it was Depo-Provera.)

Secondly, there does seem to have been a small but disturbing

A Low Sperm Count

Unfortunately, vast numbers of men do have a low sperm count (or no sperm at all) even though they're perfectly capable, virile lovers.

That's why the simple, inexpensive test of doing a sperm count should be carried out very, very early in the investigation of a couple with infertility problems (and certainly long before the woman is subjected to any uncomfortable, expensive or time-consuming tests).

All the man has to do is to provide a sample of his seminal fluid in a hospital specimen jar. He should climax directly into the container and not, as many men do, in a condom – because the rubber may harm the sperm.

The specimen jar should be taken within an hour or two to the hospital laboratory, where it will be examined under a microscope and a count made of the number of sperm in it. Repeat tests are often necessary, mainly to exclude technical errors.

Why is the sperm count so often found to be low? The sad answer is that in most cases we simply don't know.

Sometimes a man's sperm output is low (or even zero) because of past infection of the testicles – particularly by mumps. Sometimes it's low because of injury to the testicles, or because of a recent spell of ill-health. Also, certain drugs can depress sperm production, as can some hor-

SPERM COUNT

tendency for a few white doctors to regard it as an acceptable way of controlling black fertility for so-called 'sociological' reasons. In one notorious case in Britain, a doctor gave a black woman the Shot while she was under a general anaesthetic (and therefore somewhat unlikely to give her consent); his rather unusual justification for this was that he had done it in the interests of the taxpayers.

On the other hand, I have to say that the Shot is a very effective contraceptive, which is actively *demanded* by a small number of women for whom no other method is suitable. Its chief known side-effect is menstrual chaos. Any woman who opts to use the Shot must understand that her periods may become very frequent, or disappear.

---

mone disorders. However, very often the cause remains a mystery.

Treatment

If the sperm count is repeatedly *nil*, then I am afraid that there is usually little that can be done. The couple should consider AID (Donor Insemination) or adoption.

However, if the sperm count is merely on the low side, then there *is* hope. You'll get detailed advice from your infertility clinic, but possible ways of improving the sperm count include:

wearing loose, cotton underwear instead of tight, synthetic-material briefs (the latter increase the temperature of the testicles, and this depresses sperm production)

having surgical treatment for any *varicose veins* which may be present just above the testicle (a common condition)

having hormone treatment to stimulate the testicle – though this method is of very limited success

'saving up' love-making – in other words, abstaining from sex for a week or so before the woman's ovulation day, in order to build up the sperm count.

SPERM COUNT • THE SPONGE

Q I have one child, but after trying for three years for another one, we found that my husband's sperm count is low. The hospital advised him to dip his testicles into cold water before intercourse. This is rather chilly on the bottom! Is there anything else we can do to increase his sperm count?

A Well, for a start I'm afraid that there's no point in carrying out this somewhat masochistic ritual *immediately* before love-making, as sperms take about six weeks to mature inside the male body. So, as far as anybody knows, the 'cold water treatment' will only improve your man's sperm count in about 42 days' time. But wearing cool, unrestricting underpants certainly is important.

Another useful measure was revealed in a recent paper in *The Lancet*. Three Australian doctors say that if you get a man really excited, and give him plenty of love-play before intercourse, then he'll produce more sperms. They got this idea from the world of agriculture, where, they state, it's well known that 'preliminary teasing of a bull results in samples of better quality'!

The Sponge

The Today Sponge (sold in some countries under the name 'Prelude Sponge' or 'Collatex Sponge') came onto the market in various countries, including the UK and the USA, in the mid-1980s. It's a vaginal sponge, and the interesting thing about it is that it is very acceptable aesthetically to many women who appreciate its non-messy qualities.

It's a soft disc of sponge, about 5 cm (2 in) across. The sponge comes already impregnated with spermicide, so you don't have to add any when you want to make love.

All you do, in fact, is to take the Today Sponge out of its pack, moisten it, and then gently tuck it into the topmost part of your vagina — using the tips of your index and middle fingers to ensure it fits tightly against the cervix. Neither you nor your partner should be able to feel it during intercourse.

The sponge has to be left in place for at least six hours after intercourse, though it can be left in for up to two days if necessary. When the time comes to remove it, you simply hook your finger round a polyester tape which is attached to the underside.

STERILITY

The Today Sponge is disposable, and you can buy it over the counter in a chemist's shop (without a doctor's prescription).

But how safe is the Today Sponge? There have been claims that it is 98% effective. But anyone who has studied the history of contraception knows that claims like that nearly always need to be taken with a generous pinch of salt.

Ms Walli Bounds of London's Margaret Pyke Centre, who is probably the UK's leading expert on intra-vaginal contraceptives, is sceptical of the figures which have been put forward. She warns that the true failure rate of the Today Sponge may well turn out to be higher than that of any of the reliable methods which are widely used at the moment, such as the cap.

In the USA, a New York congressman has claimed that the Today device may cause cancer. But the US National Institute of Health flatly denies these allegations, and the FDA itself has given its approval for the device to go on sale.

There have also been suggestions that the sponge could cause the dangerous Toxic Shock Syndrome (the overwhelming infection which is usually associated with tampon use). But so far I know of no cases in Britain.

Sterility

About 10 to 15% of marriages have trouble with fertility. Inability to have children is a very distressing problem for any couple. Of course, not everyone can expect to have children exactly whenever they want them, but if you've been trying for, say, 12 months without success, then it's as well to seek help.

The family doctor will usually refer patients to a gynaecologist who specializes in the treatment of infertility; many hospitals run (badly overcrowded) infertility clinics these days. Alternatively, simple tests are often done at Family Planning Clinics.

At these clinics, the first problem is sometimes found to be that the wife is still a virgin and the couple are not really having intercourse at all! This may sound astonishing, but even in these supposedly well-informed days there are a surprising number of husbands and wives who simply don't know how to set about having a child (though they usually think that whatever they are doing is how babies are made).

Assuming that this problem does not apply, however, the next thing is to decide whether the couple are trying at the right

STERILITY

time of the month – *i.e.* ovulation, which is usually about 14 days before the start of a period. If you have intercourse each day for three or four days running at about the time of ovulation, then the chances of pregnancy are much better.

If this fails, full investigation of both parties is necessary. Even today, men tend to blame infertility on women, but the fact is that in many marriages it's the husband who is sterile, even though he may be potent or indeed highly virile.

The gynaecologist will therefore arrange a lab test on the husband's seminal fluid, mainly to see how many sperms it contains, and if the individual sperms are active and normally formed.

A post-coital test is also useful. The woman is examined shortly after intercourse, and a check is made as to whether the husband's sperms are surviving in the secretions of the vagina and cervix.

The woman also needs full investigation, of course. She may have to have a D and C (dilatation and curettage), or scrape of the womb lining. Very often, the specialist will test whether her Fallopian tubes (which carry the eggs, or ova, from the ovaries to the womb) are blocked or not. This is checked by a simple procedure in which a little carbon dioxide gas is blown through the tubes from a narrow catheter inserted into the vagina. X-rays of the tubes can be carried out by injecting a radio-opaque dye in the same way.

Both these procedures are more comfortable under general anaesthesia, but they can also be performed without an anaesthetic. And the technique of laparoscopy (in which a slim telescope-like device is used to

Sterilisation

In most western countries (and many developing ones) the use of sterilisation, both female and male, has increased dramatically in recent years. A very large number of couples are choosing sterilisation once they have completed their families.

As for female sterilisation, the first thing to understand is what it does. The point of the operation is to block the woman's Fallopian tubes in some way, so that the sperm cannot get to the ovum.

This can be done by cutting

STERILISATION

inspect the internal organs) can be of great help in investigating infertility. An ultrasound 'scan' of the lady's ovaries may also be helpful.

Treatment

If some disorder of the female genital tract is present, it can often be treated satisfactorily, and pregnancy may follow within a few months. If the Fallopian tubes are blocked, however, there may be a considerable problem, though some surgeons are beginning to achieve encouraging results with Fallopian-tube surgery.

And of course, the British pioneers and others all over the world have engineered the births of thousands of 'test-tube babies' – babies who are conceived in a laboratory dish from the husband's sperm and the wife's 'egg' or ovum. The fertilised ovum is then put into the womb *from below* – thereby by-passing the diseased or missing tube. The newer 'G.I.F.T.' technique involves placing sperms and an ovum in the wife's Fallopian tube.

In many cases of female infertility, particularly those linked with hormone imbalance, the new 'fertility drugs' may be very helpful.

When infertility is due to the husband, the outlook is not usually very hopeful, though there are ways of raising low sperm counts. If there is no prospect of his fathering a child, he and his wife should consider whether they want to have a baby by AID (artificial insemination by donor). An increasing number of gynaecologists are willing to arrange this procedure, and couples who have chosen it are usually very happy with their baby.

---

through the tubes and tying them off, or by clipping them with a device like a very firm plastic paperclip. The effectiveness of sterilisation is very *nearly* 100%, but, as with any operation, occasional failures do occur.

The two common methods of carrying out the procedure are:

traditional sterilisation

laparoscopic sterilisation.

'Traditional' sterilisation requires a longer stay in hospital. It's done through an incision – perhaps 10 or 13 cm (4 or 5

STERILISATION

ins) long – in the lower part of the abdomen, round about the top of the bikini line.

Laparoscopic sterilisation is the newer and much more minor operation. It's done with the aid of the slim, telescope-like viewing device called the laparoscope. This is pushed through a very tiny incision near the navel, while a 'tube-clipping' instrument is pushed through another very small incision in the woman's side.

Quite obviously, most women would prefer to have this newer operation, but it's not available everywhere in the world; not all women are suitable for it; and there is a slightly higher failure rate (i.e. pregnancy rate) than with traditional sterilisation.

Q I'm thinking of getting sterilised. Is it true it can have masculinising effects?

A Nope. Sterilisation is a simple piece of 'plumbing work' on your tubes. So it shouldn't have any hormonal effects, or put hair on your chest. There have been suggestions that it can make the periods a bit heavier, but so far there's no proof of this.

Syphilis

The most serious of the venereal diseases – apart, of course, from AIDS. Fortunately, it's rare nowadays in Britain, and other types of VD (for instance, gonorrhoea and NSU) are much more frequently encountered. Promiscuous homosexuals are at risk, however.

Syphilis is caused by a germ called *Treponema pallidum*. It can always be cured, if it's caught in the early stages. If it's not properly treated, however, the long-term consequences (which include insanity and death) are quite horrifying. Fortunately such late complications rarely occur these days, partly because most people go to a 'Special Clinic' as soon as the symptoms appear. A few patients are still unwise enough to think that the disease will go away by itself – but it won't.

Symptoms

Syphilis is acquired by having sex (though not necessarily actual intercourse) with an infected person. (*N.B.* In many countries, though not in all, there is a very high risk of infection in

SYPHILIS

having sex with prostitutes.) Very occasionally, a person with a syphilis sore on the lip may infect others simply by kissing.

The first symptom occurs nine to 90 days after exposure. A firm, painless sore develops on the genitals (or sometimes on other parts of the body, *e.g.* the lip or nipple). In women, there is a danger that the sore may sometimes be too far inside to be noticed.

The sore is usually smaller than your fingernail. A small amount of discharge may come from it. The nearby groin glands will probably swell up. After a variable period of time, the sore will go away. This does not mean the disease is cured – it isn't.

In the secondary stage of syphilis, which is usually a few weeks later, there may be a spell of general ill health, with sore throat, skin rashes, mouth ulcers and fever.

The tertiary (late) stage of syphilis occurs years later. Its appalling effects on the brain, heart and other organs need not be described here. These complications will *not* occur if you have sought treatment in the early stages of the disease.

Treatment and Prevention

Patients are sometimes tempted to treat themselves with 'borrowed' drugs because they are embarrassed about going to the doctor, but this is foolish – treatment is a specialised business. If it is to be adequate, proper lab tests have to be carried out.

In order to obtain these tests, you really need to attend the confidential Genito-Urinary Medicine Clinic (that's the new name for 'Special Clinic') at your nearest large hospital. You will probably be given a course of treatment lasting approximately two weeks, and it's vital that you don't abandon it part of the way through. You'll also be asked to return for further tests at a later date, and you'll be given printed cards to hand or send to anyone you have slept with.

Anyone who has syphilis (or any other form of VD) should on no account have sex with anybody until they are cured.

TAMPONS • TESTICLES

Q I'm going on a nudist holiday with my daughter this summer and we both want to know what ladies do about 'sanpro'.

Little strings or pads ruin poolside elegance. How do naturists cope?

A Quite easily, ma'am. Menstruating naturist women wear bikini bottoms or shorts.

The fact is not generally known,

The Testicles

It's fairly important for a woman to have a working knowledge of the male testicle – if only because it's so awfully easy for her to hurt it in bed! So be careful where you put your knees . . .

The testicle (also known as the testis) is an incredibly pain-sensitive part of the male body. This fact is vital to remember if you're *attacked* by a man. If at all possible, hit him as hard as you can in the testicles – and then run, because the disability is only temporary!

The testicle is, of course, the source of the millions of tiny sperm whose aim in life is to unite with a ripe ovum from the woman's ovary and so form a baby. Sperm, which are pro-

TAMPONS • TESTICLES

simply because 'nudist' magazines prefer, for some reason, to print pictures of people who are totally naked. Also, some naturist ladies tuck the little blue string just inside.

Q I lost a testicle when I was young, but am now happily married, with a good sex life and two children.

However, I feel that I am living with a deformity, and I would very much like to 'stand up and be counted' with other men! So, could I have an operation to put in a 'dummy' testicle?

A Yes, though you wouldn't get it on the NHS. The cost would be considerable, and there'd be an additional charge for the plastic prosthesis, which feels and looks very much like a real 'ball'.

As with any operation (especially

---

duced by the testicle, find their way up through a man's 'plumbing' in order to be ejaculated at the moment of climax. Anything up to 500 million of these are produced in a single orgasm.

But what actually happens to the testicles as a man gets sexually excited? Well, they're drawn upwards so that they press hard against his body. The work of Johnson and Masters indicates that if his testes do *not* do this, then he probably won't reach orgasm.

The two testicles have another function, which is to produce the male sex hormones, which give the secondary male sex characteristics of hairiness, muscularity, aggression, and so on.

Each testicle is rather like a flattened ping-pong ball in shape and size. Average dimensions are about (4 cm) (1¾ ins) long, 3 cm (1¼ ins) deep, and 2½ cm (1 in) thick.

Testicles occasionally have to be removed because of accident or disease. These days it's possible to replace a lost testis with a plastic one, which feels very like the real thing.

Although testicles are pain-sensitive, men do like them to be held by women – but gently! You shouldn't actually rub your partner's testicles; but if you hold them gently – particularly during intercourse – you'll find he'll appreciate it.

TEST-TUBE BABIES

a rather unusual one) you should weigh up the risks of something going wrong before you finally choose to go ahead.

Q I have appalling thrush, and all my doctor treats it with is an interminable course of Nystatin, which is messy and stains my pants orange. Isn't there any other treatment?

A Yup, there is, ma'am. Nystatin is actually a good, reliable remedy, but you have to use it for 14 days — and, as you rightly say, it does have the unfortunate 'side-effect' of staining your knickers an unpleasant colour.

Here are some other drugs which are available and which can be used just as a single dose of one vaginal tablet: Canesten 1;

Test-tube Babies

The test-tube baby technique is one of the most brilliant medical advances of recent years. It has now enabled well over 1,000 childless women to have the babies they so much wanted.

Invented by two determined and clever men, British researchers Dr Robert Edwards and the late Patrick Steptoe, the technique is basically an ingenious way of getting round the all-too-common problem of blocked tubes.

It's important to realize that it isn't usually of help with other causes of infertility, as people often think.

The Steptoe technique is really a method of bypassing the blocked tube. The surgeon removes a ripe ovum from the woman's ovary, using a telescope-like device known as the laparoscope.

Then the ovum is incubated in a glass dish, along with sperm provided by the husband. One of the sperm fertilises the ovum — and not long after the fertilised ovum is inserted into the woman's womb, via a slim tube passed up through her vagina.

Remember, however, that at present the technique is very expensive. Furthermore, at the moment only a minority of attempts succeed. If you're paying for each attempt, you could ruin yourself financially.

Still, it's undoubtedly a great step forward in combating infertility. (By the way, the 'test-tube baby technique' is something of a misnomer, since at no stage is a test tube involved in any way.)

THRUSH

Thrush

This is by far the most common vaginal infection in most countries. It's a fungus which causes:

intense soreness of the vagina

itching

an annoying discharge, which is usually creamy white.

In men, thrush usually produces no symptoms, but some men become red and sore. However, the sex partner of a woman with thrush is very possibly *carrying* it. Both partners should use an anti-fungal cream, and she should also use anti-fungal pessaries (vaginal tablets).

If thrush keeps recurring, your urine should be checked for diabetes. Thrush is more common in diabetics, and some diabetic males have to be circumcised if it keeps giving them trouble.

If you think you have thrush, you should go to a doctor and have a vaginal swab taken, to confirm the diagnosis. The doctor will usually give you both anti-fungus cream for your exterior surfaces, and anti-fungus pessaries (vaginal tablets) to clear things up inside.

If you've read what I said above about hygiene, you'll appreciate that you should also avoid: tights, nylon pants, hot baths, *men* – at least until the condition is cured!

In recurrent cases, Pill-users may have to consider switching to another contraceptive.

Note: if you develop thrush, this does *not* mean that your partner – or indeed you – have been unfaithful.

Ecostatin-1; Gyno-Daktarin 1; Gyno-Pevaryl 1.

Also, you can now take oral tablets for severe thrush: these include Nizoral and the newly released Diflucan.

And don't forget the practical anti-thrush measures: avoid hot baths; don't wear knickers; avoid promiscuous blokes; make your man use an anti-thrush cream – or else give him a liberal local application of yogurt!

Q You recently said in SHE that yogurt could be used as a last resort in treating thrush. But is it harmful to get it into the vagina? And is it safer to stick to natural

TIPPED WOMB • TRICHOMONAS VAGINALIS

yogurt, rather than the fruit-flavoured kind?

A It's quite safe to put yogurt into your vagina as a treatment for thrush, though it's quite tricky to do. But I don't think you should use the fruit-flavoured kinds, because they tend to have all sorts of odd particles in them.

Indeed, about ten years ago I remember being summoned by an agitated family planning nurse to view a patient who had 'red specks all over her cervix, doctor!' Of course, the lady had been filling herself up with raspberry yogurt – and the 'specks' were the pips.

Q I suffer from a 'tipped womb' which I believe a lot of other women have too. Is it true that there's some special position in which it would be easier for me to conceive a baby?

A Yup. Women with 'tipped' (that is, retroverted) wombs are as common as left-handed ones. It just means that the womb points in a backwards direction instead of forwards.

If you're retroverted and having trouble in conceiving, then it's a proven fact (albeit a little-known one) that the best position to use when making love is kneeling on the bed with your bottom stuck up in the air.

I suppose that's what you'd call a hot tip. Good luck!

Q You have in the past stated that *Trichomonas vaginalis* can be transferred to women by men. But how on earth does the *man* get treated?

A Well, *Trichomonas vaginalis* (TV) is the second commonest cause of vaginal discharge, after thrush. It does go back and forth between women and men, in ping-pong fashion. So the male should *always* be treated as well, even though he won't usually have any symptoms.

Regrettably, often the husband/boyfriend doesn't get treated – with the result that the woman keeps on getting the discharge back again.

So any woman who is diagnosed as having TV should ask the doctor for Flagyl (or similar) tablets to give to her partner – and make him take them! Doctors may be unwilling to prescribe Flagyl if male partners are not on their list – so in that case, blokes must go to their own doc.

VAGINA

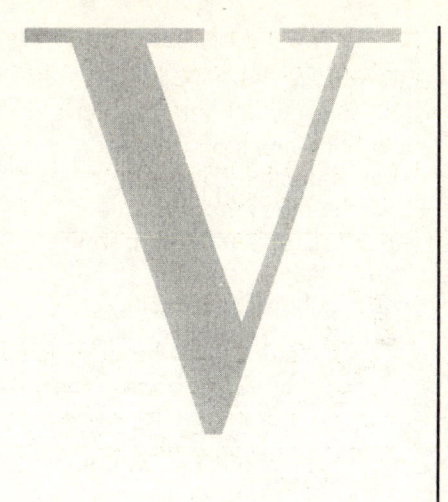

Vagina

The vagina, or 'front passage' as it's often quaintly called, is the wide, spacious, moist and well-cushioned channel which leads from the exterior up to the neck of the womb.

The word 'vagina' is Latin for 'sheath', and the reason for the name is of course the fact that the vagina provides an ideal 'sheath' for the penis.

There are many disorders of the vagina, and some of them can be extremely distressing for a woman. In this particular sphere, far too many patients suffer in silence. If you have some sort of vaginal trouble, the golden rule is to go and see your doctor before things get any worse. Don't delay because of embarrassment. The doctor will examine you and, if necessary, order lab tests or send you to see a gynaecologist. Family Planning Clinics provide another source of advice, as do Well Woman clinics.

Vaginal bleeding

Any type of vaginal bleeding other than the blood loss associated with completely regular periods needs assessment by a doctor.
BLEEDING DURING PERIODS (MENSTRUATION). Heavy

VAGINA

menstrual blood loss ('flooding') and irregular menstruation can readily cause anaemia, and should be treated as soon as possible.

BLEEDING BETWEEN PERIODS. Intermenstrual bleeding or bleeding after intercourse (even if it's only 'spotting' on the underclothes) may be a serious symptom. A full gynaecological examination is advisable. See your doctor within two or three days. But 'spotting' can also be due to an inappropriate brand of Pill (and is normal during the first couple of months on the Pill).

BLEEDING AFTER THE MENOPAUSE. This too may be a serious symptom and needs immediate gynaecological assessment. Again, consult your doctor at the earliest possible date.

BLEEDING IN PREGNANCY. In early pregnancy (up to five months), bleeding is usually due to a threatened or actual miscarriage. In late pregnancy, bleeding may be due to various causes, but must always be reported to your doc.

Vaginal and Pelvic Infections

These are so common that the great majority of young (and not so young) women these days get them at some time or other. These infections do seem to have become much more frequent since the advent of the permissive society.

That's hardly surprising, because it seems likely that all of them can be spread by sex – at least some of the time. Other factors which have made vaginal infections so much more common in the last 30 years are:

wearing tights (some organisms – especially thrush – *love* the warm conditions under a pair of tights)

wearing nylon underwear (same effect)

the fashion for frequent hot baths and Jacuzzis (which also promote hot, moist conditions)

the widespread use of the Pill (which seems to make you more liable to thrush)

the widespread use of antibiotics (which also promote thrush)

Fortunately, most vaginal infections aren't serious – though they can be an irritating nuisance and badly mess up your sex life!

However, *deeper* pelvic infections – which attack the tubes – can be very serious, and can

VAGINA

even make you infertile. This is in fact a common cause of infertility today.

Vaginal Irritation and Discharge

IRRITATION. Vaginal irritation usually occurs together with discharge (but see also PRURITUS).
DISCHARGE. One of the commonest of all symptoms, and one that causes a great deal of worry – often unnecessary worry.

It's important to stress that, from puberty onwards, a certain amount of vaginal secretion is completely normal. A lot of teenage girls don't realise this. Because they're often embarrassed about consulting their own doctors, they deluge newspaper and magazine advice columns with letters about this problem!

The vaginal fluid should be thin and reasonably clear; it has a natural aroma, the presence of which does not indicate a need for the use of douches or vaginal deodorants. The rate of secretion of the fluid varies from time to time and increases markedly when sexually aroused.

So when does a discharge need medical attention? Basically if it's thick, if it's yellow, green, brown or red, if it's irritant or associated with soreness or pain, or if it smells offensive.

Causes of discharge include disorders of the cervix (neck of the womb), and particularly cervicitis, cervical erosion and cervical polyps. Other common causes are infection by thrush and by the trichomonas parasite.

It's worth knowing that lately we've discovered that certain 'new germs' can cause vaginal discharge. A very common one is called *Gardnerella vaginalis*, which causes a greyish discharge with an embarrassing smell. It's treatable with Flagyl tablets. Also, never forget that a forgotten tampon can be a cause of vaginal discharge.

If you have one of the types of discharge outlined above, see your doctor. He should examine you and may send swabs to the lab for examination. If necessary, he should arrange an appointment with a gynaecologist.

Most types of vaginal discharge and irritation respond promptly to adequate treatment, though recurrences may occur in some cases. In view of the recent emergence of 'new' vaginal infections (like Herpes), if in doubt don't hesitate to go to a 'Special' or 'Genito-Urinary', clinic.

VAGINA

Q I am a teenage virgin. For some years I have had vaginal discharge, but my doctor doesn't seem to know what to do about it. Is there anywhere else I could go?

A Yes – there's a branch of the Brook Advisory Service for young people in your city: have a look in the phone book. But if you're a virgin, it's unlikely that there is any very serious cause for this symptom. (Most cases of serious infection are, I'm afraid, caused by sex.)

Q For over a year now, I've suffered with an extremely smelly vaginal discharge. Every swab and smear my doctor has taken has been negative, so I am at my wits' end.

A Sorry to hear about this. My best suggestion is as follows:

Quite often, an offensive discharge is caused by anaerobes, common germs which may not show up on conventional tests. It's characteristic of these organisms that they produce a distinct smell, which is offensive to the woman and (less frequently) noticeable to her partner.

Fortunately, anaerobes can be done in by oral tablets called Flagyl. An alternative is to use Flagyl *pessaries*, to be inserted into the vagina every other day.

Offensive discharge caused by anaerobes is common, and the fact that Flagyl cures it is not all that well known. In fact, recently I heard of a case in which a woman who'd had a very trying, offensive discharge for many years was only cured when by pure chance her dentist prescribed Flagyl for an anaerobic infection of her gums.

Q I have a fishy smelling discharge of the type which you mentioned in SHE earlier this year.

I was delighted when I read your article, because you said it could be treated with a tablet called Flagyl. (My GP had been unsuccessfully trying to treat it with antibiotics.) When I told him about the article, he gave me Flagyl, which cured the discharge.

But now it's come back again. Is this connected with the fact that I've been unfaithful to my husband? I'm afraid I dare not tell my GP this.

A Well, yes; you may well have been re-infected, either by your husband or by your lover.

I want to stress that Flagyl (also known as metronidazole) is *not* a cure-all for every type of vaginal

VAGINA

discharge. Nor will it take away the slightly fishy smell, which — for many women — is both healthy and normal.

I don't know what your doc actually diagnosed. But if you really feel that you can't go back and tell him the truth about your sex life, then I reckon you should go instead for a confidential chat and check up at a Genito-Urinary clinic.

Q For a long time, I've been extremely bothered by adverts for vaginal products which contain local anaesthetic.

I have always been led to understand that use of a local anaesthetic in this area could result in becoming sensitive to such things. Isn't that so?

A Yes, I'm afraid you're right. Local anaesthetic is used in some commercial preparations — with the specific idea of 'numbing' vaginal irritation or soreness.

Expert gynaecological opinion is against the use of these products — because (fairly obviously) if you've got something wrong with your vagina, you need to get it treated, not anaesthetised!

Also, you're quite right in saying that the application of a local anaesthetic can occasionally result in extremely painful sensitivity reactions.

Q I have recently been treated with Flagyl for a vaginal infection, presumably trichomonas.

But my husband has simply refused to take the same tablets, because he says 'he would know if *he* had any infection'. Would he?

A How remarkably silly of him. As I keep saying in SHE, women who have this common vaginal infection are all too liable to get it back again *if their sexual partners don't take the pills too.*

Tell your husband that men who carry trichomonas *don't* have symptoms. I think you'd be very unwise to have sex with him till he's agreed to take the tablets.

Q I hope to go water-skiing this summer. But is it really true that there are some special dangers for women?

A I fear so. There have been a number of cases in which the jet of water coming up from the ski has penetrated the woman's vagina, and caused serious injuries.

Nor is it just the women who're at risk: there's been at least one case of a chap who got a nasty squirt up his bottom and had to

VAGINA

spend some time in hospital recovering.

However, I'm told that there is virtually *no* danger if you wear a proper protective wet-suit, with the usual strap underneath. But under no circumstances should anyone go water-skiing in a bikini — or (as I believe sometimes occurs among the jet set) in the nude. This is asking for what us doctors call 'trouble down below'.

Q After four children, my vagina is terribly loose, so that love-making is not as satisfying as it should be. I can't face the thought of a repair operation (which you mentioned recently in SHE), so what can I do?

A I must have had hundreds of letters recently about laxness of the vagina. (I hasten to add that when I speak of vaginal laxity, I mean the muscular, rather than the moral variety.)

Here are two useful tips for readers who find that their vaginas have become a little slack: (1) Try making love with your thighs *together*; this helps you to grip your man much more firmly; (2) If your bloke is fairly adventurous, get him to experiment with gently putting a finger inside you *at the same time as he's making love to you*; this simple technique gives you a lot more 'bulk' inside a loose vagina.

Q My vaginal muscles have been slack since the children were born, and this is affecting our love-making.

I know you have mentioned exercises to get these muscles back to normal. Can you recommend any literature which explains these? Also, is there a self-help group for women with this problem, which I believe is common?

A It sure is, ma'am! In fact, my postbag is full of letters on this subject.

Many gyms and women's aerobics classes now offer a course of pelvic floor muscle re-education. The basic exercises are explained on page 94. By the way, I recently encountered a journalist who asked me if pelvic floor exercises were so called because you did them on the floor!

Q Some friends invited my husband and me to a nude party in their indoor swimming pool. Things got a bit out of hand, and I made love with several guys in the water. What I am worried about is,

VAS DEFERENS

could the chlorine in the pool have damaged my vagina?

A I'm assuming this letter isn't a hoax – since I see it was posted in the Surrey stockbroker belt, where sex in the swimming pool seems to be as socially acceptable as smoked salmon and Sainsbury's Soave.

I'd have said that chlorine is the least of your problems – for I know of no evidence that it damages a woman's innards. But if you go on having orgies in the indoor pool, you are in some danger of (a) pregnancy of unknown origin; (b) drowning.

The Vas Deferens

The *vas deferens* is the tube which brings sperms up from the testicle towards the penis. A man normally has two of these tubes: a few blokes have three, but this *isn't* an advantage to them, as we'll see in a moment.

The *vas* looks very like a thin piece of spaghetti. It can be felt with the fingertips through the skin of a man's scrotum (gently, please!) as – it runs up towards the groin.

But the reason why there's such a lot of interest in the *vas* these days is that it's the bit they chop when they do vasectomies.

This fantastically popular operation just involves making two tiny incisions in the skin of the scrotum – and then working via them to cut through each *vas*, and then tie the ends off.

Why are men who have a third *vas* at a disadvantage? Because the surgeon probably won't realise they have an extra *vas deferens*, and will fail to cut it. So, in their cases, the vasectomy won't work!

Happily, the sperm test which is done a couple of months or so after a vasectomy will detect the fact that there's another *vas deferens*, still sending up vast supplies of spermatozoa. The third *vas* can then be cut and tied off too.

Cutting through the *vas deferens* doesn't interfere with a man's production of sex hormones, or with his virility. It just gives him a great feeling of confidence that he's no longer exposing his female partner to the risk of unwanted pregnancy.

And that, of course, can make a *vas deferens* to his love life . . .

VASECTOMY

Vasectomy

While I was preparing this book, I was a bit disturbed to read that vasectomy had just been declared a crime in Italy. Yes – it's now a criminal offence, for both surgeon *and* patient! Presumably tourists with vasectomies will still be allowed in: at least, I hope so – because I happen to have had one.

In most civilised countries, however (especially those where the *machismo* tradition is dying), vasectomy has become fantastically popular in recent years. Surgeons find it hard to keep up with the demand, and it has almost become a matter of routine for the younger middle-aged man to consider getting himself vasectomised, to spare his wife the health risks of more years on the Pill or the IUD.

Among medical families in Britain, a recent study showed that about a quarter now rely on either vasectomy or female sterilisation as their method of contraception (with a 50/50 split between the two methods).

A vasectomy is really a very simple business indeed – and far less complex and traumatic than female sterilisation because the 'plumbing' is all external. The operation is often done under local anaesthetic – and indeed, I watched my own being done (though I wouldn't recommend this to the faint hearted).

In the few days after the operation the man can expect a fair amount of bruising and swelling. He should wear a support, and may need to take some pain-killers. He should definitely *not* undertake any heavy work (lifting, etc.) for several days.

There are a few complications, such as the occasional stitch slipping, leading to bleeding or a large but temporary swelling. Inevitably, this happened to *me* – and I had to spend about three weeks in bed. For full horrendous details, see Dr Richard Gordon's best-seller *Great Medical Disasters* (London: Heinemann Books).

But I've never known anybody come to any long-term harm

Q My sister's baby died after her husband had a vasectomy. What are his chances of reversing it?

A I'm so sorry to hear about this. Your brother-in-law's best bet would be to see the consultant urologist at a Medical School.

VASECTOMY

from a vasectomy. Unusually for surgical operations, no deaths have *ever* been reported —except for two tragic cases of lockjaw, which occurred in two men who were operated on in insanitary conditions in India.

Happily, a couple can resume love-making as soon as they like after the operation (some have been known to manage it about 2½ hours afterwards!). The man will not be 'safe', however, until he has had – on average – about a dozen climaxes, to clear out all the sperm in the upper part of his piping.

Surgeons recommend a simple sperm test, usually carried out two or three months after the operation, to make sure that no sperm is left in the fluid. Until then, the couple should use another method of contraception.

Yes, there *is* fluid produced – effectively the same volume as before. And yes – sex is just as good afterwards as it was previously.

However, men with psycho-sexual problems should be screened out by the counselling sessions provided before a vasectomy – partly because a man who has deep fears of castration may mistakenly get the idea that the operation has lessened his potency, or affected him in other ways.

Finally, if as a couple you decide on this method, there is one other thing you should bear in mind. It is this: *do not go in for it if you think you might change your mind.*

In general, it is best to regard vasectomy as an irreversible step. There *is* an operation to reverse it, but the results are not very good. So both of you should be very sure that vasectomy is the right *permanent solution to the question of contraception in your relationship.*

Note: No operation has a 100% success rate, and there are very rare cases in which a man fathers a child long after an apparently successful vasectomy.

He may be willing to attempt a reversal. But the 'pregnancy rate' is often well below 50%.

Because the results of vasectomy reversal are so unimpressive, couples who are contemplating having hubby sterilised should bear in mind that it is possible to take out 'insurance' by depositing sperm in a private sperm bank.

VASECTOMY

Q My husband had a vasectomy some years ago, and we have made love without any protection since then. But he says that he has recently read reports of vasectomies failing after many years – and women getting pregnant as a result. Is this true?

A Well, nothing (including vasectomy) is ever 100% effective. It's true that there have been recent headlines about surgeons getting into trouble for failing to warn men about this ('Top Docs Face Sex Rap').

Every male who has a vasectomy should have one or (preferably) two sperm tests a few months after the operation, to make sure that he's not fertile. If this is done, then the couple can assume that the chance of further sperms finding their way through the bloke's blocked-up plumbing is fairly remote.

In practice, there's a general feeling that many (if not most) pregnancies which occur after a vasectomy are due to the well-known 'Milkman Syndrome'.

Q My husband is having trouble in getting a vasectomy because our doctor is violently opposed to anyone having the operation. Could we get it done privately?

A Certainly. There are now many private surgeons and clinics who do this astonishingly popular op. For instance, your husband could talk to the Marie Stopes Clinic in London (01-388 2585), which has always specialised in low-cost vasectomies. (I had my own done there.) It's a snip at about £100!

Q My husband had a vasectomy about 12 years ago, toward the end of his first marriage. After his divorce, he met me and we got married and have enjoyed a good relationship ever since. Would there be any chance of reversing the vasectomy, so that we could have children of our own?

A The chances of successful vasectomy reversal are not great, I'm afraid. But some intrepid surgeons – particularly in teaching hospitals – *are* willing to have a bash at this difficult and challenging operation.

The type of surgeon you and your husband need to consult is a urologist. They're a bit thin on the ground, but as it happens there is one at the large hospital in the town from which you write.

VENEREAL DISEASE

Venereal Diseases

VD is common nowadays, particularly among young adults. Anyone who has had a casual sexual liaison would be well advised to go to a hospital 'Genito-Urinary Clinic' for a check-up, *under conditions of strict confidentiality*. A few simple tests carried out there will tell whether infection has taken place. (These clinics are advertised quite widely nowadays. If you're in doubt, ring the nearest large hospital and enquire when the next 'Special Clinic' will be held, or call the Family Planning Information Service at 01-636 7866.)

It's important to bear in mind that VD in women (and occasionally men) may well produce no obvious symptoms. Therefore, if you have the least suspicion of it, have a check at once. Treatment, if carried out right away, is usually curative.

Prevention

VD is virtually always passed on by having sexual contact (though not necessarily actual intercourse) with an infected person. Repeated contact is not necessary – a few seconds can give it to you.

It's obvious, therefore, that VD would be rapidly wiped out in a world in which everybody was always faithful to his or her sexual partner. Blatant promiscuity, or 'sleeping around', is very likely to lead to infection, particularly in cities, large towns, and ports, where the incidence of VD is always high. Unfortunately, 'new' infections like herpes and AIDS are beginning to spread alarmingly in such areas.

In Britain, and some other countries, it's been shown statistically that a man who goes with street prostitutes is virtually certain to get VD before long.

Wearing a sheath and washing carefully immediately after intercourse provides at least some protection against venereal infection, but not much; it's far more sensible to avoid 'sleeping around'.

If you suspect that infection has occurred, cease all sexual activity at once in case you spread the disease further. If the clinic finds that you actually *do* have VD, you'll probably be given tracing slips to give to anyone you've slept with recently. Though it's embarrassing, always pass these on: otherwise the consequences for these people (and their future sexual contacts) may be disastrous.

VIRGINITY · THE VULVA

Q I live in the Arabian Gulf, and a friend of mine is desperate to have her virginity restored by the operation you recently mentioned in SHE. My friend gave her virginity to the boy she loved at age 16. But now she must be a virgin in order to be married.

We are visiting England soon, and she could have the operation then. But you have said that there are some incompetent plastic surgeons in Britain. So who should she contact? Please help — you're our last hope.

A Your 'friend' wouldn't happen to be yourself love, would it?

Anyway, I think that the best thing to do would be to write to the British Association of Aesthetic Plastic Surgeons, c/o The Royal College of Surgeons, *35, Lincoln's Inn Fields, London WC2*. The operation is expensive. But I hope it will achieve the desired effect on the wedding night.

Q I read what you wrote in SHE about how women shouldn't feel that their vulvas were ugly or abnormal. Well, I'm not happy about the appearance of *mine*, because the labia are far too long.

I would like to get them operated on before the summer holidays. Is this possible?

A What sort of summer holidays are you going on, I ask myself! Well ma'am, you'd have to get your skates on in order to have your labia shortened by bikini-time, but it can be done.

Though I honestly wouldn't recommend this op for most people, I am told by a cosmetic surgeon that there is a procedure which is known in the plastic surgery trade as a 'fanny-plasty'. It costs around a thousand quid, and it's possible to get it done through the British Association of Aesthetic Plastic Cosmetic Surgeons, mentioned left.

Please note that I *cannot* guarantee the results of such an operation to re-shape your vulva, though I quite understand your reasons for asking about it. After all, as Keats says in *Endymion*, 'A thing of beauty is a joy for ever...'

Q I feel that my sex organs are terribly ugly because my labia minora project through the labia majora.

I am too embarrassed to go to the doctor about this, but could I pos-

THE VULVA

sibly have an operation to put it right?

A The recent Delvin Report survey showed that quite a high proportion of women are unhappy about the appearance of their vulvas.

From your very clear and concise description I think you may actually be *normal*, but if you're badly distressed about the way you look, then certainly an operation is possible.

The vulva 'tidying-up' op usually costs somewhere in the region of a £1,000 surgeon's fee, plus hospital charges for your stay.

I really do think you should go to your doc's straight away and let him/her have a look at you to see if the operation is a reasonable idea to give you peace of mind.

Q I'm 43 and have recently developed a curious lump on the side of my vulva. My husband wants me to go to the doctor, but surely this isn't necessary?

A I beg you to have this checked out *immediately*. Unexplained lumps or ulcers on the vulva – particularly in the over-40s – demand an urgent medical opinion.

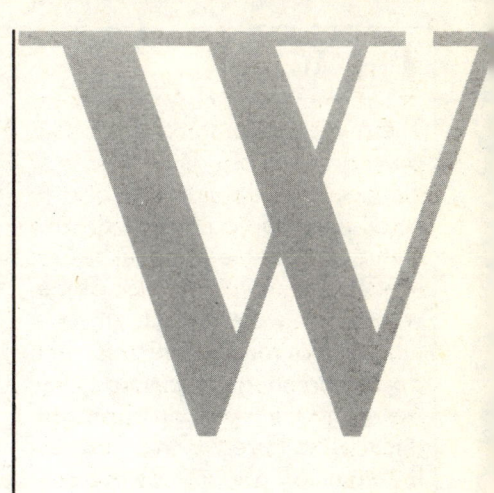

THE WOMB

The Womb

The average woman's womb is only about as big as her clenched fist. It's very like a small pear, turned upside down, with the tip of the pear representing the cervix, or neck of the womb. The womb is actually a little bag of muscle which is powerful enough to push a baby out – and it's the contraction of this muscle fibre which produces the pains of labour. However, the womb is not all muscle. There's a thin lining, which is shed every month when a woman has her period.

Disorders

There are very many disorders of the womb. This is one reason for the fact that about one out of every five women eventually has her womb removed.

The main disorders are:

Fibroids. Benign swellings which develop in the muscular wall. Incredibly common, particularly in the over-thirties and in women who haven't had children. The cause is unknown and the symptoms are pain, or heavy periods, or difficulty in passing urine. If they don't cause symptoms, they can usually be left alone. Troublesome fibroids may have to be 'shelled out' or a hysterectomy may be necessary.

Prolapse. Prolapse of the womb means that it comes down into the vagina, and may even come outside. It's caused by weakening of the supports of the womb during childbirth. It is curable by a repair operation, or if necessary a hysterectomy.

Endometriosis. Painful nodules in the wall of the womb, and elsewhere in the pelvis. Treatable with hormones or, if necessary, surgical removal.

Cancer of the womb lining. Womb cancer (which is quite different from cancer of the cervix) kills about 1,000 British women each year. It usually starts in the womb lining, and can be triggered off by excessive stimulation with oestrogens. This is most common in women who have passed the menopause – and the giveaway symptom is *bleeding occurring after the menopause*. This must *always* be investigated. Cure is possible by hysterectomy.

Unfortunately, there is as yet no widely available screening test for cancer of the womb. Smear tests (for cancer of the cervix) do *not* detect cancer of the womb. There is a test, called 'out-patient curettage', but at the moment cost prevents it from being widely used.

Useful Addresses

General Health and Information

Cancer Relief
Anchor House
15–19 Britten Street
London SW3 3TZ
Ph 01–351–7811

Haemophilia Society
123 Westminster Bridge Road
London SE1 7HR
Ph 01–928–2020

Herpes Association
Omnibus
41 North Road
London N7
Ph 01–609–9061

Institute of Psycho-Sexual Medicine
11 Chandos Street
London W1M 9DE
Ph 01–580–0631

British Association for Counselling
37A Sheep Street
Rugby
Warwickshire CV21 3BX
Ph 0788–78328

National Council for Civil Liberties
21 Tabard Street
London SE1 2LA
Ph 01–403–3888

Release
169 Commercial Avenue
London E1 6BW
Ph 01–377–5905
24-hour emergency line 01–603–8654

Health Education Council
Hamilton House
Mabledon Place
London WC1H 9TX
Ph 01–631–0930

Cosmetic and Plastic Surgery

British Association of Aesthetic Plastic Surgeons
c/o The Royal College of Surgeons
35 Lincoln's Inn Fields
London WC2A 3PN
Ph 01–831–5161

Gay/Homosexual

Albany Trust Counselling
24 Chester Square
London SW9 9JF
Ph 01–730–5871

Gay Switchboard:
BM Switchboard
London WC1N 3XX
Ph 01–837–7324

Terence Higgins Trust
BM Aids
London WC1N 3XX
Ph 01–831–0330

Family Planning

Natural Family Planning Clinic
Birmingham Maternity Hospital
Queen Elizabeth Medical Centre
Birmingham B15 2TG
Ph 021–472–1377

Pregnancy Advisory Service
11–13 Charlotte Street
London W1P 1HD
Ph 01–637–8962

Family Planning Association
27–35 Mortimer Street
London W1N 7RJ
Ph 01–646–7866

British Pregnancy Advisory Service
Austy Manor
Wootton Wawen
Solihull
West Midlands B95 6BX
Ph 05642-3225

Brook Advisory Centre for Young People
153A East Street
London SE17 2SD
Ph 01-708-1234

Marie Stopes Memorial Clinic
108 Whitfield Street
London W1P 6BE
Ph 01-388-0662

National Childbirth Trust (NCT)
Alexandra House
Oldham Terrace
London W3 6MH
Ph 01-992-8637

Birth Centre (London)
101 Tufnell Park Road
London N7

La Leche League
BM 3424
London WC1 6XX

Miscarriage Association
PO Box 24
Ossett
Wakefield
W Yorkshire WF3 3DD
Ph 0924-830-515

Marriage

RELATE (National Marriage Guidance Council)
Herbert Gray College
Little Church Street
Rugby
Warwickshire CV21 3AP
Ph 0788-73241

Association of Sexual and Marital Therapists
c/o Dr L Webster
St Mary's Hospital
Hathersage Road
Manchester M13 0JH
Ph 061-276-1234

Women's Health

Breast Care and Mastectomy Association
26A Harrison Street
London WC1H 8JG
Ph 01-837-0908

Women's National Cancer Control Campaign (WNCCC)
1 South Audley Street
London W1Y 5DQ
Ph 01-499-7532

Endometriosis Society
65 Holmdene Avenue
Herne Hill
London SE24 9LD

Women's Aid Federation
52-54 Featherstone Street
London EC1

Rape Crisis Centre
PO Box 69
London WC1
Ph 24 hr line 01-837-1600

Children

Incest Crisis Line 01-422-5100

Association for Postnatal Depression
7 Gowan Avenue
Fulham
London SW6

Parents Anonymous for Distressed Parents
6 Manor Gardens
London N7
Ph 01-263-8918

National Society for the Prevention of Cruelty to Children
67 Saffron Hill
London EC1N 8RS
Ph 01–242–1626

Single Parent Families

Gingerbread
35 Wellington Street
London WC2
Ph 01–240–0953

National Council for One-Parent Families
255 Kentish Town Road
London NW5 2LX
Ph 01–267–1361

Adoption

Parent to Parent Information on Adoption Society
Lower Boddington
Daventry
Northants NN11 6YB
Ph 0327–60295

National Association for the Childless
Birmingham Settlement
318 Summer Lane
Birmingham B19 3RL
Ph 021–359–4887

British Agencies for Adoption and Fostering
11 Southwark Street
London SE1 1RQ
Ph 01–407–8800

Parents for Children
222 Camden High Street
London NW1 8QR